THE ACTOR'S SECRET

THE ACTOR'S
SECRET

Techniques for Transforming Habitual Patterns and Improving Performance

BETSY POLATIN

North Atlantic Books
Berkeley, California

Published by
North Atlantic Books
Berkeley, California

Cover and book design by Brad Greene
Printed in the United States of America

The Actor's Secret: Techniques for Transforming Habitual Patterns and Improving Performance is sponsored and published by the Society for the Study of Native Arts and Sciences (dba North Atlantic Books), an educational nonprofit based in Berkeley, California, that collaborates with partners to develop cross-cultural perspectives, nurture holistic views of art, science, the humanities, and healing, and seed personal and global transformation by publishing work on the relationship of body, spirit, and nature.

North Atlantic Books' publications are available through most bookstores. For further information, visit our website at www.northatlanticbooks.com or call 800-733-3000.

MEDICAL DISCLAIMER: The following information is intended for general information purposes only. Individuals should always see their health care provider before administering any suggestions made in this book. Any application of the material set forth in the following pages is at the reader's discretion and is his or her sole responsibility.

Library of Congress Cataloging-in-Publication Data

Polatin, Betsy.
   The actor's secret : techniques for transforming habitual patterns and improving performance / Betsy Polatin.
       pages cm
   Summary: "The Actor's Secret is comprised of explorations and exercises developed from the Alexander Technique, a practical method for self-improvement and neuromuscular reeducation; Breathing Coordination, an approach that increases breathing capacity and awareness; and Somatic Experiencing, the body-based approach to healing trauma."
   ISBN 978-1-58394-682-4 (pbk.) — ISBN 978-1-58394-683-1
   1. Acting—Study and teaching. 2. Alexander technique. I. Title.
   PN2075.P64 2013
   792.02'807—dc23   2013014090

                    3 4 5 6 7 8 VERSA 21 20 19 18

*This book is dedicated to those who have the courage
and willingness to pursue change in themselves.*

ACKNOWLEDGMENTS

I am very grateful to the teachers, mentors, and guides who have shared their wealth of knowledge with me over the years. This knowledge has come through books, hands-on experience, sensory feedback, deep inquiry, and observation. I am grateful to the pioneering innovators of somatic work, who had the courage to explore the unity of body, mind, and spirit. Thank you to those visionaries who encouraged me to learn and teach this work.

The exercises in this book are a synthesis of my physical, mental, and spiritual training throughout my life of learning from many fine teachers. My teachings and exercises have been influenced by F. M. Alexander, Carl Stough, Peter Levine, Rivka Cohen, Patrick Mac-Donald, Marjory Barlow, Frank Pierce Jones, Helen Jones, Tommy Thompson, David Gorman, Rob MacDonald, Margaret Goldie, Pedro de Alcantara, Kelly McEvenue, David Garlick, Frances Cott, Richard Schwartz, Jessica Wolf, John Baron, Deirdre Fay, Raja Selvam, Diane Poole-Heller, Bessel van der Kolk, and spiritual and meditation teachers. Many, many thanks to all.

A very special thanks to Boston University's College of Fine Arts School of Theater faculty, my wonderfully skilled colleagues whom I have the pleasure of working with on a daily basis. Much love and appreciation to all my students whose lives I have had the privilege of sharing. A special thank-you to Harry Miller Hobbs II, Clifton Dunn, Dayna Cousins, Ben Thompson, Liza Burns, Hannah Burkhauser, and the entire Boston University School of Theater acting class of 2010, for demonstrating the exercises in the photos in this book.

Thank you to Chia Messina, photographer, for capturing a wonderful moment for the back page photo. Thank you to Ion Sokhos, photographer, for taking all the beautiful photos in the book. Thank you to Nina Ryan for her clever and insightful editing and for her early encouragement and interest in the book. Thank you to Janet Banks for reading a draft and telling me, "You have a winner." Thank you to Daria Polatin for contributing her superb writing and editing skills, which, combined with her knowledge and understanding of my work, helped create a more seamless read. A very heartfelt thank-you to North Atlantic Books and my editor, Jessica Sevey, for taking on this book. Thank you to copy editor Christopher Church, and to the designer of the book cover and interior, Brad Greene.

Thank you to all my loving friends and family for their unending support and encouragement, especially to Daria and Ruby, my daughters.

CONTENTS

About *The Actor's Secret*

After my first Alexander lesson, I walked out of the room thinking, "This is still me, but not the me I always knew. Actually, a very different me than I knew when I walked in." This brief experience of an altered sense of self excited and daunted me at the same time. I had moved through an opening, pulled aside an inner veil, and been exposed to radical new possibilities and choices of how I sensed myself and saw the world around me. My body felt less constricted, my mind was less worried, and my senses were more vibrant and alive. The colors of the world seemed brighter. As I walked along the street that day, I knew I was still me, but a different me: a new me.

I have continued exploring and teaching this experience of an expanded self through a unique combination of approaches. In my forty years of teaching and coaching, I have witnessed many students discover their habits and feel their way through their own veils of delusion and resistance into new worlds of artistic choice and experience. One successful woman I taught said after a lesson, "I thought I had all there was to have in life." On the surface, she did. She had a successful career, a good family, money, friends, and happiness. But after studying with me in hands-on sessions, she said, "I see there is so much more to life that I didn't even know about: aspects of myself I had no idea existed."

Actors express their version of the same idea. "I thought I understood this role, but when I stopped doing what I was sure was so right, the performance opened up in a way I never imagined." This book is written for you, the actor, who is able to lose his or her own habitual identity and become another person in behavior, body, voice, and being. Actors transform themselves to tell a story while an audience watches. In performance, every word, gesture, and movement of an actor tells a piece of the story to the audience. Even with a natural ability and imagination for this kind of transformation, most actors need coaching, guidance, options, and tools to meet the challenges of acting with full awareness. An actor asks the questions, "Do I believe I have full body, mind, and spirit living in the life of this play?" "Do I believe wholeheartedly what I am saying and doing?" Do my body movements accurately convey the situation?" "Am I willing not to know what happens next?" "Am I present and aware?" If the answer to any of these questions is no, something needs attention. This book provides many opportunities for an actor to expand his or her awareness, and it can lead to positive changes in acting and everyday life.

The Actor's Secret comprises explorations and exercises that I have developed mainly from the Alexander Technique; Breathing Coordination, the work of breathing expert Carl Stough; and Somatic Experiencing, the trauma work of Dr. Peter A. Levine. I bring together these three different techniques to help you explore your own path of discovery to the experience of an expanded self. This unique combination of approaches provides revolutionary new training and resources for the actor.

The Alexander Technique is a practical method for self-improvement and neuromuscular reeducation. Breathing Coordination is a method for increasing breathing capacity and awareness. Somatic Experiencing is a way of working through traumas, big or small, by a process that includes tracking bodily sensations to restore well-being and healthy functioning. These three techniques address how we "use" ourselves, or how we use our body, mind, and spirit to do what we do. We either close and constrict or open and expand our channels of expression. The unique combination of Alexander Technique, Breathing Coordination, and Somatic Experiencing that my work is made up of can give you the ability to open your channels of expression so that you can say "yes" to the above questions and so that your work is fully embodied, both mentally and physically.

I find that many actors have a feeling or knowledge within themselves that "I can do this." They see what other actors do, and feel they have the voice, the body, and the creative imagination to do that as well. But when it comes to rehearsal or performance, they often don't feel that they have performed as well as they could have. I have heard this again and again. Between the thought and belief of being able to do something and the execution of actually doing it, something gets in the way. Has this happened to you? You knew how to play a moment, but for some reason it didn't turn out the way you intended. Perhaps your body felt restricted, or your emotional connection to the character wasn't as strong as it could have been. Or perhaps your breathing was limited and your voice wasn't expressive. Or maybe you were doing similar repetitive interpretations that you always tend to do.

What is in the way? Habitual patterns are—physical and psychological habits. Habits that interfere with the manifestation of innate raw talent and skill are in the way. Habits of body tension, fear, emotional response, and survival are in the way. These habits, often formed long ago, were appropriate at that moment for your survival. For example, an individual might have a habit of smiling often in an effort to make everybody happy and create a safe environment, even though he or she is not actually happy and the situation may in fact be hostile. Are these kinds of habits appropriate now? Is it possible that some of the habits you formed to manage your life may be short-circuiting and getting in the way of your innate raw talent and skills? If you are an actor and have a habit of smiling a lot, might this interfere with playing a grave situation?

An actor needs to be present and spontaneous to be most effective on stage or screen. An actor wants to be able to access a full range of body movements and emotional expressions, from larger than life to small and subtle. Often things like inefficient breathing, vocal tightness, and unhelpful movement habits interfere with full artistic expression. This book teaches you how to become aware of those habits, and to move beyond them.

This is more than just a how-to book, explaining how to do some exercises to make you a better actor. I teach people to change by accessing their own sensory experience, which can range from a simple pain to a complex emotional state. An actor may say, "My back hurts." This back pain can interfere with the actor's ability to transform into a character that does not have back pain. In a more extreme case, an actor once came in for a lesson and told me, "I spend half my day holding back my tears." How could she expect to be fully present to transform into another character if she was dealing with such an extreme sensory experience?

The exercises in this book will help you recognize your own habitual patterns that block spontaneity and prevent you from transforming into another person. This work also develops kinesthetic and sensory awareness, which can lead to effortless coordinated movement, greater knowledge and command of breath and voice, genuine emotions, and consistent and sustained character choices that will enhance your performance.

The Actor's Secret guides you from the early stages of rehearsal to the final performance. It gives you the tools and techniques necessary to experiment and to discover a vibrant and commanding performance. When you have an awareness of yourself, the ground beneath you, your breathing, and the strength and breadth of your back, allowing you to let go of your habitual responses, you have the secret. With these skills of increased awareness and letting go of old habits, you can revolutionize your performance as you practice the age-old art form of telling a story.

My Approach

*The greatest good you can do for another is not just to share
your riches but to reveal to him his own.*
 — Benjamin Disraeli

I have always been fascinated by, and curious about, movement and
stillness in human response. How and when does the body move
in the most efficient and effortless way? How are we designed to
function and move? What are the inner hierarchies that govern our
responses, our sensory experiences, and our relationship to gravity on this planet? I have dedicated my life to exploring how the
body works and the elements of human potential, well-being, and
the performing arts. Over the past forty-five years, I have studied
in various fields, including the Alexander Technique, dance and
movement, music, acting, breathing, voice, healing arts, trauma,
meditation, and spirituality. This work has given me the ability
to help people change—to transform how they move, how they
breathe, how they perform, and how they connect with themselves
on an inner level.

The primary aspect of my work is the Alexander Technique,
which I have studied and taught for thirty-five years. In addition
to completing two three-year training courses, I have studied with
renowned Alexander Technique master teachers from all over the
globe, including many who studied directly with F. M. Alexander,
the founder and inventor of the technique. I have presented my
work to Alexander Technique experts in national and international
conferences, including one at Oxford University. I have taught the
technique in private sessions and master classes worldwide, and I
am currently the professor of the Alexander Technique in the acting
conservatory at Boston University College of Fine Arts, where I have
been teaching since 2000.

A few years into my teaching of the Alexander Technique, I
started to notice that many people still did not breathe fully. Their

lungs and ribs didn't expand to their full capacity, making for shallower breathing and less oxygen circulating in the body. I wondered what might be the most efficient way to breathe. I researched many experts on the subject, but I was not satisfied until I found the Breathing Coordination principles, the work of Carl Stough. Carl invented a series of hands-on exercises that help people improve their breathing capacity. This work helps actors as well as people with respiratory illnesses. Carl taught me his unique breathing techniques firsthand, and designated me as one of the few teachers to pass on his work. I have incorporated his breathing techniques into my work for the past twenty years.

As I continued to teach, I found that many students were still not able to make lasting changes in themselves. I wondered why. One of the avenues I explored was trauma. I read books on how the body remembers and processes overwhelming experiences, and how this affects the bodily systems. One of the most influential books that I read was *Waking the Tiger* by Dr. Peter A. Levine, a major innovator in the world of trauma. From this book I learned that many people hold patterns of trauma in their bodies from large and small challenging experiences. In many cases, years of talk therapy did not address or solve these patterns of trauma. Like other forms of habit, these deep patterns dictate our responses until they are recognized and resolved. Fifteen years ago, I was fortunate to find and train in Somatic Experiencing, Peter's experiential training course. When I studied the advanced-level courses on healing trauma with Peter, he invited me to present my work on breathing to trauma-work professionals.

My teaching also includes my life experiences. I have danced in an Andy Warhol movie about the Velvet Underground, meditated on a mountaintop in Mexico with an enlightened spiritual teacher, and traveled on five continents. These experiences have helped deepen and widen my knowledge of the world and how we live in it.

Having studied and taught the Alexander Technique, breathing, and trauma work for many years, I have designed the simple yet effective exercises in this book as a guide for you to explore and discover your own habits, and to learn to function without them, maximizing your potential for creative and personal growth. My approach is highly accessible. I believe doing is learning. The exercises here are the experience. If you pay attention to yourself with awareness and observation as you do the exercises, you will identify what is standing in the way of you reaching your higher body-mind and creative potential, and shift what is blocking you from achieving that improvement. You will understand your own "use"—the way you use your body, mind, and spirit—and begin to discover and develop your true nature and innate talent.

How to Use This Book

Because actors work on their feet a lot of the time, this book is designed to function on a three-dimensional, participatory level. The main ideas and exercises are outlined in the following way:

1. **The bold print will introduce unfamiliar vocabulary or new concepts.**
2. The standard print explains the main ideas and principles, and gives a deeper understanding of how and why you do the exercises.
3. *The italicized print is "the script." It is the subjective text for you to use as you do the exercises. You can read the script onto a recorder and, in your own voice, prepare yourself for performance.*

For an actor, the use of this book is twofold. You can learn how to use yourself well to keep your body, mind, and spirit functioning optimally. However, you can also learn how to identify patterns of use and misuse to convey the specifics of a character. Since plays are often not about people who are healthy, together individuals who use themselves well, identifying and using patterns of misuse, can be very helpful in creating the quirks and various habits of a character.

I use the word *exercise* in describing the activities in this book, but they are not the "no pain, no gain" type of exercise designed to build muscles. **The exercises contained here are explorations into your direct human experience.** The practices here are to guide you as you journey inside yourself, and they will help you understand sensations, thoughts, and micromovements that you might notice are starting to happen.

While working through the exercises, when you are asked to notice what is happening in your body, the idea is to become aware of what you are doing. The goal is not to manipulate yourself or to get rid of tension. Often these manipulations will cause even more tightness than was originally present. The goal is being aware. Cultivating the practice of awareness is a powerful tool, because once you are aware of what you are doing, you have the power of consciousness to change it.

Once you become aware of changes that are starting to happen, you have the opportunity to own them. For example, as you do an exercise, your arm may feel lighter. You may want to say, "The arm feels lighter." Instead, what we are exploring here is saying, "*My* arm feels lighter." This way you are more involved in your own process of discovery, owning yourself and being part of the process of the change that is taking place.

The exercises in this book are presented in a sequence that is helpful to an actor in rehearsal for stage or screen. That said, the exercises can also be done in any order after you have become familiar with the principles in chapters 1 to 7. The frequency of practice may vary as you need it. Some of the exercises may provide adequate information when explored once, but the warm-ups may be something you want to do regularly before rehearsals or performances. Other exercises, such as the Exercise to Explore

Lying-Down Work, can be done daily. The practice of "giving basic directions" and "can I do less" can be done multiple times a day. Once you have come to understand the principles of this book, it is up to you how you want to use the tools. Use them in whatever way best suits your needs.

The Actor's Secret contains exercises for a single person, pairs, and groups. The exercises are the core experience of the book. They are like experiments, exploring different potential aspects of your self and the characters you play. The more you explore the exercises, the deeper the unfolding can be. The photos give you some idea of what the exercises look like, and what you can look for as you practice them. Some of the photos show how a teacher can clarify the exercise. If you are not an actor, you are welcome to use the exercises in this book as a general means of self-exploration. Use what is helpful to you, however it best suits you in your profession and daily life.

As you begin your journey of exploring The Actor's Secret, allow yourself to be open and curious about unknown aspects of yourself. Remember that change occurs on many levels, and size does not equate to importance. Try to stay open to the range of shifts and changes that may be taking place, and see if you can learn and grow from those changes. Perhaps you will find your "new me."

Part One
PRINCIPLES

CHAPTER 1

What Is the Actor's Secret?

The key lies in choice. How are you sitting or standing right now? While you read these words, how do you respond physically, or emotionally? Can you feel your body weight on one foot or the other? Are you sitting leaning toward one side or the other? Are you squinting, hunching forward toward the page, leaning in against the edge of a counter or a table? Are you gripping the book tightly? Can you feel the pull of your shoulder muscles, or do your shoulders feel weightless? Can you feel sensations in your body, in your gut, in your heart? Do you have awareness of some parts of your body but not others? Are you choosing these things, or are they your habitual way of reading? Did you realize that you had the power to choose how you hold and read this book?

The key to choice lies in self-knowledge of your habits and an awareness of how you "use" yourself, or how you do what you do. Try turning the page of this book, or answer your cell phone. Do you use your right hand or your left? Do you lean your ear toward the phone, raise one shoulder while you're talking? Are you breathing fully? Do you know if this is your habitual response? Do you know you can choose to use yourself another way to answer the phone, or turn a page? The key lies in choice based on awareness of your body, mind, and self in relationship to your environment. Now, what do you think you might look like to a person across the room? Does that person see the same use of your body, mind, and self that you sense? How are we using our bodies really? How are we using our selves?

The Actor's Secret **is not talking about alignment or body positions, but about "use": how we use our whole body, mind, and spirit to do what we do.** The concept of "use" is fundamental to this book and has to do with the way we manifest and express our selves—consciously or unconsciously—in our particular habits of being. For each person these habits are unique, and each person must discover for himself or herself the patterns of their own use. Your use includes how you hold your body, how you breathe, and how you sense your internal state.

F. M. Alexander said, "Talk about a man's individuality and character: it's the way he uses himself."[1] Actors portray a variety of characters, each with very different use, just as every person uses his or her body differently. The concept of use can be seen to affect body and mind, and thus the whole self. If you as an actor are either unaware of, or unable to change, your own use, how can you transform into another character? If you have no feeling in your feet, how can you portray someone who is very grounded? Or if you feel trembling or butterflies in your stomach all the time, how can you pretend not to feel that and play a character with a calm stomach? In my teaching, the concept of use expands the opportunities for an actor to change. The following is an example of the Actor's Secret.

A student I worked with, who we'll call Carol, was playing a character with a big and generous heart. Every time she worked on her scene, she felt she could not portray the generosity and fullness that she knew her character had. Carol was trying hard to portray her character as generous, but something seemed to be in the way of her expressing that. Carol came to me for coaching and asked me to help her feel this sense of generosity in her character. I asked her to do her monologue. When she finished, I asked her, "What did you notice?" She said that she felt like she was "trying" to be generous. She also said that she often felt like she had no other choice but to try to "make" something happen. She was forcing the feeling of generosity, but it still wasn't translating as making her character seem warm-hearted. **I told her that I understood that she did not feel the generosity, and instead of trying to feel the generosity that she did not feel, I asked her what it would be like to pay attention to what she *did* feel.** After a few moments of contemplation, paying attention to what was going on in her inner state, she said she felt a tightness in her chest, as if there was a metal plate in her upper chest. I asked her to pay attention to the plate and describe it to me. She said it was a silver color, and very thick. She then said it was protecting her heart. I asked her to keep her awareness on the metal plate in her chest for a few moments. She stayed focusing her attention on this inner image of the plate, and breathed in and out calmly for a few moments.

Then I asked, "What does the plate look like now?" She said it was melting. She said that she felt sad, and she began to cry a little. Then, after feeling this metal wall around her heart melting, she exhaled a huge sigh of relief. Her ribs began to expand and contract, enabling her to breathe more fully and deeply. I encouraged her to allow her deeper breathing to continue. I then suggested that she allow her whole body to recognize and integrate the change that had taken place in her chest. The feeling of the metal plate protecting her heart was gone. Carol said "no" to her habitual pattern of trying to feel something that she did not feel (generosity), and instead she stayed with what she did feel and tracked her sensations. I asked her to do the monologue again with this new awareness of her self, and the whole room. I also asked her to feel the support of the ground beneath her, that gravity was supporting her, rather than fighting against her. As she spoke the words of the monologue again with her breath moving, her feet on the ground, and her back lengthened and widened, she was able to feel the generosity of her character and express the feelings of an open heart. She felt lighter in her chest, and she was not trying to make anything happen—it was just happening. She was able to say "no" to her habitual pattern. Thus her "use" changed. She was using her body, mind, and spirit in a new and more productive way.

This example of an actor's process demonstrates a few main elements of my work. When an actor comes in to work with me, I have the actor present a piece that he or she is working on or having difficulty with. I then ask, "What did you notice?" From there, the investigation begins. The actor and I explore how to access and change personal habitual patterns, so that the actor can transform into the character.

In the case of Carol, the Alexander Technique gave her inner direction, support, and expanded awareness. Breathing Coordination gave her the ability to expand her ribs, letting them move freely on her spine and sternum, and thus have a more complete and fuller breath. Somatic Experiencing, the body awareness approach to trauma, gave her the experience of tracking her bodily sensations. This allowed her to feel her actual sensations rather than work to override them. As Carol's nervous system settled, the autonomic branch of the system was able to self-regulate, normalizing her bodily functions of breathing and heart rate. *The Actor's Secret* explains these components and gives you exercises to explore them. These explorations can lead you to more choice. Then you too can say "no" to your habitual patterns and choose to use yourself another way. The following chapter provides a brief overview of the techniques.

CHAPTER 2

Innovators of Three Somatic Techniques

Many years ago as a young dancer, I loved the feeling of moving through space, feeling my whole body in motion. But I was not interested in just moving on stage and making sure my choreography and body looked good; I also grew curious about how bodies moved in general, and without causing injury.

I used to go to the ballet in New York City with my dance teacher, Frances Cott. Frances called what she did "technical dance analysis." We sat in the second balcony and watched the dancers on stage. Every once in a while she would poke me and say, "She is going to fall off that pirouette" (a ballet turn with one leg raised). I waited in awe to see if she was right. She always was. She could analyze the muscle pulls and see where the dancer's movement pattern was leading. If you pull muscles in one direction, your whole body is moved in that direction. If you pull muscles in another direction, they move you another way. The body has a hard-wired organization for movement. Frances understood this. I studied with Frances for many years to learn this type of movement analysis, and started to understand how the body operates most efficiently and with no pain.

Because actors have only their bodies to tell the story of the character and the play, it is crucial for them to understand how the body works most efficiently. Many acting studios refer to the body as "the instrument." The instrument includes every aspect:

body, mind, emotion, spirit, and more. An actor must learn to use this instrument well. My lifelong work is to continue to discover how the body-mind-self works most effectively and efficiently. The people in the following three stories share with me this overwhelming interest. We have in common the curiosity of how the body takes in, interprets, and remembers: how it works, how it doesn't work, how it is designed to function, how it functions best, how the biology is organized, and how to change. I, and the people in these stories, have all sorted out use in one way or another.

Introduction to the Alexander Technique

In my first Alexander Technique lesson, as I mentioned in the Introduction, I was struck by the change that had occurred within myself. With the expanded awareness I experienced after my lesson, I tuned in to an overall awareness of an organization of my body that was deeper than anything I had ever felt. This deep, all-inclusive organization of my body-mind-self seemed to be a universal force that was larger than me, global in nature, and could be beneficial to the whole human race. **It was not just a muscular framework for a dancer to move well and not fall off turns, but a force that seemed to me to be a necessary component of evolution and the survival of all creatures.** I wondered if this was the internal organization that survived millions of years of change. Maybe it was the organization that allows a two-thousand-pound polar bear to jump over a cliff as if he weighed practically nothing?

The teachings of Frederick Matthias Alexander form part of the foundation of my work. I tell Alexander's story for three reasons. First, he was an actor, so his story has special significance for this book because his discovery of the Technique came directly out of his work as an actor. Second, the story of how he developed his technique teaches us the qualities of observation and awareness that led Alexander to insights about the way we use ourselves. Third,

Alexander's story illuminates the profound effects of his willingness to experiment, to see and observe with his own eyes, mind, and spirit, and to persist in his ideas and exploration.

Born in Australia in 1869, Alexander was a well-known elocutionist, specializing in Shakespearean recitation. He developed a one-man show of Shakespeare's great soliloquies that he toured and performed. Early in his career, Alexander began losing his voice during and after performances. He tried a number of medicines and cures, and finally was told by his doctor that he had to stop performing if he wanted to save his voice. However, Alexander noticed that in daily conversation he had no problem with his voice. His voice only failed when he performed. He wondered if it was possible to observe what he was doing while performing that was causing his voice to shut down. If he could discover what he was doing and stop doing it, perhaps he could recover his voice.

This approach to the problem of losing his voice while performing led Alexander to a very important idea, which he later called "use," meaning how we use ourselves, taking into consideration our whole self—body, mind, and spirit. He then began to study how, in his terms, "use affects function"—meaning that how we use our selves, or what we do with our selves, determines how we function. One of my acting students read this part of Alexander's story and commented, "I never would have thought that my vocal trouble was something that I was doing. I would have blamed the theater, the acoustics, and everything else."

Driven by the desire to continue acting, Alexander spent the next ten years exploring the possibilities of his misuse and experimenting with ways to change. Through observation and awareness, Alexander discovered the cause of his vocal trouble. By watching himself in the mirror, he observed that merely the thought of reciting triggered a pattern of what he called "misuse," beginning with the head. Alexander noticed that when he was reciting, he pulled his head back and down, which depressed his larynx. With these interferences went a tendency to suck in breath, lift his chest, and hollow his back, thus shortening his stature. This was Alexander's misuse. As he began to teach his technique to others, he realized that many actors had similar misuse habits.

You would think misuse could be solved simply by "not doing" the actions that cause problems, and by "doing" something else. But solving misuse is not always as simple as it may seem. As Alexander was discovering, what we think we are doing and what we are actually doing are often two different things. Usually when something is wrong, we think we must do something to fix the problem. But Alexander realized that doing "more" only tangled him more. Doing more is a common habit with actors, especially when they are trying to convince the audience of something. Leaning forward, for instance, so that the audience will "get it" or tightening muscles more to show anger are common tendencies. The solution that Alexander found was first to stop responding to his problems in his habitual way.

Alexander found that he was able to maintain good use until the last second before speaking or making a movement. At that moment, he reverted to his familiar and comfortable use, which is to say, misuse. This is a critical moment—the space between the stimulus to respond (in Alexander's case, to speak) and the response—the space within which the possibility of freedom from habit is most likely to occur. At this moment you have a choice to react in the habitual way, or to respond in a new way. Here, within this moment, is where Alexander's concept of inhibition came into play. He used the term "inhibition" in a positive sense. **By inhibition he meant delaying the instantaneous response to a stimulus; withholding consent to automatic reaction to allow a response that maintains the cohesive action of the whole organism.** He believed that any movement or response not generated by the coordinated integrative action of the nervous system would cause problems. Learning to allow this moment of freedom opens the door to an integrated response. This is what I call the Actor's Secret.

Alexander continued to teach this technique that he developed for many years in London, where he died in 1955. Alexander's books explain his process of discovery and his philosophy. They do not contain exercises, as the Alexander Technique does not have a specific set of exercises. In *The Actor's Secret,* I have put his ideas and discoveries into exploration form, which I am calling exercises.

The Alexander Technique is widely used by many outstanding actors and performers. One well-known student of the technique, stage and screen actor Ian McKellen, said, "I was very enthusiastic about the value of the Alexander Technique, and I made it possible for all members of the *Richard III* and the *King Lear* companies to have lessons whilst rehearsing."[1] The basic principles of the Alexander Technique are taught in this book, but if you want to continue to pursue learning about the technique, there is a wealth of information in Alexander's own writing, or you may also want to seek the guidance of a professional Alexander Technique teacher for hands-on lessons.

Introduction to Breathing Coordination

Because of my interest in movement and my years of dance training, my early years of teaching the Alexander Technique were devoted mainly to dancers through the Sports Medicine Clinic at Children's Hospital in Boston, under the direction of Lyle Micheli, MD. Then, in 1985, I was asked to teach a workshop to singers at Berklee College of Music. This immediately opened my curiosity of voice and sound to the body and movement work I had been specializing in. I started to wonder: how does the way you use your body affect the sound you produce? I began to work with many performers and explore: if you stand or move your body one way or another, what is the effect on your voice? If the muscles in your chest drop, what happens to the sound? Of course, you cannot investigate vocal sound very long without wondering about breathing. This drew me to Carl Stough. His work led me to explore breathing, sound, and movement in relation to the Alexander Technique principles that I was teaching, and also awakened my own desire to breathe and sing fully. He wrote, "Breathing is a process which will occur of itself, but proper breathing requires considerably more attention."[2] Stough was a major innovator in the field of breathing research. He was a singer who graduated from Westminster Choir College and went on to become a choir director who was widely recognized for his extraordinary ability to teach people of all ages very quickly to sing well.

In 1958 doctors from a local hospital, who were researching the then-new disease emphysema, sought his help. They thought that since Carl could teach people to sing that he must know something about breathing. At first he wanted no part of working with sick people, but after some coaxing, he decided to try to help these people with respiratory illness. **This led to his discovery of what he called Breathing Coordination, changing the use of one's breathing pattern.** Through the rest of his career, Carl worked with people with respiratory illness as well as with singers and actors. The principles of breathing coordination that Stough developed can help increase vital lung capacity, oxygenation, and vocal range, and can decrease symptoms of stress and respiratory illness, including asthma and emphysema. Breathing Coordination allows the respiratory system to function at maximum efficiency with minimum effort.

He wrote, "Every physical and emotional problem, to some degree, is the result of an insufficiency of oxygen."[3] To understand Carl's breathing coordination principles, it's helpful to start with how the breathing mechanism works. A breath is initiated when the respiratory center of your brain, which monitors blood gases, determines that you need oxygen. The brain then sends signals through the phrenic nerve, which runs from the base of the brain down to the diaphragm, to trigger the process that includes a springlike quality of movement in the respiratory mechanism. The phrenic nerve is the only motor nerve that connects to the diaphragm.

The diaphragm, one of the largest muscles in the body, is a large dome-shaped structure. Carl called the diaphragm a muscle-organ because it functions as both. To get an idea of what it looks like, imagine a grapefruit cut in half with the pulp scooped out. The diaphragm resembles the shell that is left. This dome-like shell fits up under your ribs, and the rim attaches all around to your bottom ribs like an open umbrella inside your torso. The diaphragm regulates the delicate balance of pressure above and below it. Because there are no voluntary motor nerves to the diaphragm, you are not able to voluntarily move or control your diaphragm. You can move the voluntary muscles around it, the intercostals and abdominals. These muscles influence the diaphragm, but you cannot move the actual diaphragm with your motor nerves or by your will.

As you breathe in, the diaphragm moves down via the signal from the phrenic nerve. As you breathe out, the diaphragm moves up. The up-and-down distance the diaphragm travels is called the excursion. Maximum excursion of the diaphragm is four and a half inches of motion. Even though it is possible for the diaphragm to rise and fall four and a half inches, most people have no more than one and a half inches of motion.[4] This means that most people do not use their full breathing capacity; they only use about one-third. The exercises in the chapter on breathing will help you increase your breathing capacity. As an actor, the quality and quantity of your breath can make the difference between an inspired, vocally connected performance and a flat, forced performance.

Introduction to Somatic Experiencing

As I was teaching Alexander Technique and Breathing Coordination, working with all kinds of performers, I understood more and more how the body is designed to function, and how the breath is properly coordinated. But something was still missing in completing the process of fully understanding body-mind, movement, and function. Something was off. As I watched an actor on stage, there was often a gesture, tone, or action that I did not necessarily believe. I often noticed habitual patterns that interfered with total freedom of expression—freedom to transform into another character or freedom to be present in the here and now. These observations led me to discover the world of trauma.

The majority of my trauma studies were based on theories developed by Dr. Peter Levine, a major innovator in the world of trauma detection, analysis, and healing. Levine has contributed to the research and understanding of the nature of stress and overwhelming life experiences. This somatic (from the Greek *soma*, meaning "relating to the body") approach applied to acting has been an extraordinarily powerful tool. Levine was interested in how humans are affected by stress. He studied animals in the wild. He observed that they are traumatized all the time, but they rarely have lasting or debilitating effects from the encounters. After many years of study, he concluded that **trauma is a biological process. It is a series of steps that take place physiologically, and all the steps need to be completed for full recovery from the event.**

You can see these steps demonstrated in the animal world. A rabbit is happily eating grass when all of a sudden it is attacked by a coyote. The rabbit runs away and manages to get to safety. The rabbit has mobilized his defensive responses (fight, flight, or freeze). In this case, he uses flight to run away. There is a tremendous amount of energy needed to run for his survival. The running itself uses much energy, but there is often some energy that continues to pump after the event is over and has not been used. That extra energy is still coursing through his body. The rabbit now needs to complete that step of the response in his body, and use that extra energy. So the rabbit will now lie down and tremble and shake to discharge the energy and complete the defensive response.

This same mechanism operates in humans in a similar way, but most humans respond in a different way. Let's say a woman is riding her bicycle to work, and her tire hits a rock, causing her to take a tumble. Her body mobilizes energy in her arms and legs to try to save herself. She is in a dangerous situation, so that fight, flight, or freeze response is automatically initiated by her system. As she lies on the ground, the mobilized energy that wanted to save her is coursing through her body and wanting to discharge. But what happens? She remembers that she has an important meeting that she needs to get to. Her neocortex overrides the need to discharge that extra energy, and she gets up, says she's fine (even though she is not actually fine), and goes to work. That undischarged energy remains in her system and can later show up as some kind of "random" symptom, like not being able to sleep, being overly sensitive, or not being able to focus. The techniques used in Somatic Experiencing help identify these blocks of residual energy that lie dormant in the body and manifest themselves as symptoms.

According to Levine, "Trauma lives in the body, not the event."[5] Trauma is part of everyone's life. Usually, life goes along with a flow of happenings. We have moments that are slightly overwhelming, which trigger an activation of extra energy, or slightly disappointing, which can result in a depression or dampening down of energy; we are able to recover from both. But in certain instances, unexpected, overwhelming, and horrific things happen: you trip, fall out of a tree, have a car accident, or your dog dies, among any number of other instances. All of these events leave some trace of imbalance or repetitive patterns in your body and influence your life, behavior, and choices, most of the time unconsciously. The overwhelming nature of the event is too strong to handle, so the nervous system gets thrown off balance into high activation, low depression, or sometimes both. At this point, the survival of the system has been threatened, so the defensive responses come into play. As we see with the bicycle accident, the defense response's inappropriately used energy stays in play and manifests as symptoms until the response is complete.

When the defensive response is actually complete, the body begins to self-regulate, or bring itself to a state of equilibrium. The exercises and explorations in this book can help you learn to track your bodily sensations and discover some of your deeper held patterns that may have been caused by traumatic events, large or small. Uncovering these patterns can lead you to complete these transactions and return to equilibrium. Most of the exercises do not ask you to recall the details of the specific traumas that may have caused these patterns. Instead, we will be using the process to describe the current sensations and feelings in the body. However, if an incident does arise in your explorations that is physically or psychologically upsetting to you, use your judgment and seek professional help if you need it. This work may have therapeutic effects, but it is not meant as a replacement for any kind of therapy.

Each of these three techniques highlights a different aspect of use and body functioning. They all recognize a habitual pattern or problem and offer a means of change. This is the Actor's Secret: recognizing a habitual pattern, saying no, and allowing something else to occur. Plasticity—change—is built into the process of evolving. When you understand how to improve your use, your breathing coordination, and your nervous system's self-regulation, you are then able to transform seamlessly into the character of your choice.

CHAPTER 3
Use and Misuse

The principle of "use" is not about how one specific part of the body moves. Body parts do not move independently of one another; the whole self is involved. When you stand leaning on one leg, your whole body responds: Your head tilts to one side, one shoulder drops, you exert more pressure into one heel. But when you use yourself well to walk, not leaning or pulling on certain bones and muscle groups, your body is toned, your mind is clear, and your emotions are calm. Use is an orchestrated activity of your whole self. The parts make up the whole, and a part reflects the whole.

There is a basic distinction between "use" and "misuse." Good use allows us to use ourselves in empowering ways that open and expand channels of expression, so that each movement and gesture becomes a conscious manifestation of full spirit, mind, and body. Misuse blocks, constricts, and confuses expression. **The first step in your process of discovery of an expanded self is to begin to become aware of, and learn to recognize, your own patterns of use and misuse.** For example: I tend to use myself well when I am content, or attentive. I tend to misuse myself when I am rushing, or preoccupied, or upset. Another way to describe use and misuse might be that the response to the act of rushing is often accompanied by use that is constricted and pulled in, which is considered misuse.

When I started to learn the Alexander Technique, I was surprised to discover my own misuse. I realized that I had been pulling down in my torso, and I had very little sense of contact with the ground. The pulling-down shortened my height, decreased my ability to breathe, and put pressure on the joints in my legs. I had no idea that any of this was happening before my introduction to the Alexander Technique. Because I was unaware, I had no choice about my use.

Over the years, I have worked with many students who have had similar misperceptions. Most people are limited in their options of use. Either they slump down in what is called "relaxed," or they stiffen up in what is called "good posture." (Later in the book we will discuss a third option, called "direction.") There is a common misuse associated with good posture or "standing up straight." Most people interpret standing up straight as pulling your shoulders back and lifting your chest. Neither of these actions are a good solution to the overall habit of slumping down. When you lift your chest in front, you do it by pulling down in your upper back. This compresses your upper back and does not let your whole back lengthen or widen for a more upright stance, which can offer greater ease of movement and breath.

It is important here to remember the concept of wholeness. If you have a problem with your arm, obviously you want to heal it. The common choice is to do something to "fix" your arm, like exercises or stretching. But in truth, for lasting results, you need to look at the whole picture. Your arm is about ten percent of your whole body. When your arm hurts, you are using your whole body to function as one unit in concert with your ailing arm. If you just repair your arm, the rest of your body, ninety percent, is still operating as it was with your arm problem. It is more than likely that problems will continue to emerge until you address your overall use of your entire body.

Think again about what you are doing now, as you read this page. As you read you may be thinking, "I'm not doing anything while I am reading." But you are using yourself in a specific way. Maybe you are leaning on your elbows and hunching your shoulders forward, or pulling your forehead downward. Take a moment and become aware again: what is your use as you read these words? How are you using yourself? How are you responding to what you are reading? Crossing one leg, leaning to one side, gripping your jaw, and lifting your shoulders are all common habits that are a response to reading or many other activities. Many positions, or ways of holding yourself, are possible. None are bad, per se. We are not trying to get rid of anything. We are trying to have more options as a choice of response. Habits are our response to life situations. Repetitive patterns of use can become problematic or painful when they are unconscious, or when they are done very often because they are the only choice you are aware of.

Use takes many forms: the way the body is shaped (hunched or upright), how it is aligned in space, the favored muscular pulls (leaning to one side), how body parts are positioned in relation to one another, the qualities of movement that have left an imprint through frequent repetition, how we hold ourselves at rest, inner attitudes, slight muscular holdings, and "sets." **What I call a "set" is a preparation to do an activity, an attitude of expectancy, that facilitates a learned response.** Sets may be appropriate or suited to the activity or not. A common set is to hunch over as you read, or to throw your head back as you begin to speak.

You may not be aware of many of your own patterns, which can be so embedded and automatic that they may seem unchangeable. But as you look deeper, you can see that the possibility of change is available to you, as you develop awareness and understanding of how you are using yourself. For example, holding your breath is a common pattern. You may think, "That's just the way I breathe. My breath doesn't really flow." On the surface it seems like your breath is not flowing in and out. But if you look more closely, you may see that your ribs are not moving as much as they could be, blocking your breath from flowing in and out. Becoming aware of the holding of your ribs, and choosing not to hold your ribs anymore, will allow your ribs to move, letting your breath flow in and out more freely. While nonflowing breath might have seemed unchangeable, and "just the way you breathe," now it has become a choice to let go of the holding in your ribs, allowing breath to flow freely in and out, allowing more oxygenation to take place in the body and an ease of movement in the lungs and back.

How do we begin to recognize our own use and misuse? The first step to understanding your own use and misuse is to awaken and begin using your powers of awareness and observation. I begin with misuse rather than use because, as we learned in Alexander's story, you need to understand what not to do, or inhibit, before you are free to do something else. You have to become aware of the habit before you can change it. The most common misuse is usually caused by a downward pull, often starting with the head dropping down, shortening the neck, and creating compression throughout the system. This is often accompanied by a lack of healthy postural tone, an overall slight collapse in the body. When you choose to stop pulling yourself down (misuse) you have a chance to expand upward (improved use).

The following exercises are developed from many years of coaching, teaching, mentoring, and exploring what lies at the heart of performance. The exercises are the seeds from which this book grew, and the exercises form the core experience of the book. It's helpful to practice them in a quiet space, with a mirror nearby for visual reference.

As you explore the exercises, you will embark on an active and specific journey of self-discovery: a journey to discover the universe of your own use.

Exercise to Become Aware of Common Misuse and Improved Use

Preparation: *Before you begin the exercise, take a moment just to stand. Can you feel your downward pull—a slight overall collapse in your body? Is it in your whole body, or in specific parts? Allow information from your body to come to you.*

1. *Stand in front of a mirror. Then try doing each of the common components of misuse listed below, so that you feel misuse in your body as well as see it in the mirror.*

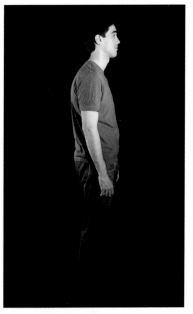

Misuse:

- *Head tilted back*
- *Neck and chin tilted forward*
- *Upper chest falling back, caving in, or sternum pushed forward*
- *Lower back arched with pelvis jutting forward*
- *Knees locked back and calves arching back*
- *Leaning forward on your toes*
- *Shoulders pulling up with inhale, dropping with exhale*

Standing with misuse.

How do you feel after exploring misuse? Do any of the movements feel familiar? Did you notice that any of these were habits of yours?

Take a few breaths, and a little walk around the room.

2. *Return to the mirror. We will now do the same process for exploring improved use. Again, try working through each of the phrases below, feeling what they do in your body and in your perception.*

Improved use:

- *Head a touch forward and up, poised on top of your spine*
- *Neck slightly back, but not overly straightened*
- *Whole back lengthened and widened, from your hip sockets to the top of your spine*
- *Weight into heels (legs unlocked), as the front of the feet spread wide on the floor*

- *Arms falling loosely by your side*
- *Ribs moving in and out with your breath*

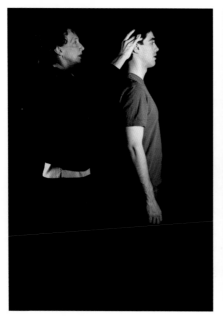 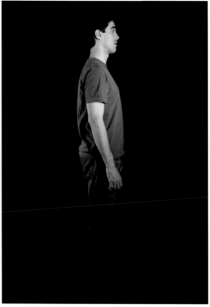

Help with improved use.   Standing with improved use.

How do you feel after exploring improved use? Does it feel familiar? Does it feel awkward? Natural? What does your shape look like in the mirror? Do you look or feel different? Often there is less physical pain with improved use.

One actor I worked with was exploring his use. He said that his neck was tight and that he often had trouble being heard. As he stood, we noticed that he was leaning forward, his weight shifted over his toes rather than his heels. He had never noticed that before. I used a gentle hands-on approach, helping show him physically how his body was leaning forward, and then gently guiding his body to lean back a little more, his weight shifting into his heels. He could now feel how his habit had been pulling him forward. When he stopped leaning forward on his own, his back lengthened and his ribs began to move in and out with his breathing. These slight physical changes of not giving in to his habit of leaning forward opened his eyes on an intellectual level, and on the emotional level as well. In his past he'd had numerous instances of feeling like he was not being heard. His body responded in a way it thought was appropriate, by leaning forward. But now, after feeling this shift of not needing to lean forward, he said, "Right now everything from the past has come into play in front of my eyes. It is really past. I feel like I don't need to go forward to get anything anymore. Because I have everything I need. I don't need to reach forward to try to be heard, and my neck feels better."

In this story, leaning forward is "misuse" in the larger picture of physical functioning, but it had been appropriate use in the past given his life circumstances of feeling like he wasn't heard. In the past, he had had to lean forward to try to get attention and to be heard, but now he realized this wasn't the case in the present, and so he was able to let go of the habit.

Exercise to Explore Your Use

1. *Stand and become aware of what you are doing in your body. For example, "I am tightening my left shoulder," or "I am holding my ribs, thus limiting my breathing," or "I am not aware of anything." Do not try to change anything, just observe.*

2. *Go to a mirror and observe what you are doing. Observe five aspects of your use in front of the mirror. Write them down in a notebook. Are you tilting your head back? Is your pelvis jutting forward? Are your knees locked? Do any of the five aspects you identified while looking in the mirror match up with what you were aware of happening in your body without the mirror?*

3. *See if you can become aware of these five aspects of your use without the visual help of the mirror. Again, don't try to change one particular part, because, remember, we function as a whole. What to do and not do about your observations will be explained later. Often when you become aware of misuse, your body immediately attempts to change it into improved use.*

This simple exploration of use can be used for any set of actions, for example, sitting and learning lines or crossing the stage. When I work with students, we often come back to this basic exercise—becoming aware of what you are doing, or how you are using yourself. While working, I often say, **"What do you notice now?"** This process of being aware of use is an important one for the actor. When you begin to see the difference between improved use and misuse, then you can choose what is helpful to you as an actor. This can be a great tool when working on a character. As Alexander said, as noted in chapter 1, "Talk about a man's individuality and character: it's the way he uses himself."

CHAPTER 4

Five Principles

There are five main principles of the Alexander Technique that can become integral to the acting process, and in general for increased body-mind awareness in daily life.

Five Principles of the Alexander Technique and How They Relate to Actors

1. The primary control
2. The power of habit
3. Inhibition
4. Faulty sensory perception
5. Direction

My approach to teaching Alexander's five basic principles emphasizes the clarity and specificity an actor can gain by using them. Using the principles, the actor can be present with increased mental awareness, a fuller voice, and a committed body. An understanding of these principles helps the actor to make choices about his or her performance, and to follow through with consistent and believable characters.

The well-known film actor Kevin Kline said, "The many benefits that the Alexander Technique afforded us as actors included minimized tension, centeredness, vocal relaxation and responsiveness, and mind-body connection."[1] The five principles explained here can provide you with the tools to gain these benefits.

1. The Primary Control

The primary control is the mechanism that governs our total pattern of coordination, the built-in system that organizes well-being, and our natural response to gravity. This mechanism governs the relationship of the head, neck, and back to the ground within the gravitational field. We call it "primary" because it comes first in every movement, and it determines the coordination and muscle tone for the rest of the body.

In all vertebrates—beings with a backbone—there is a specific relationship among the head, neck, and back: the head leads and the body follows. If your head is pulled down even a little, or forward, backward, or sideways, some kind of compression will occur underneath your head. This can show up in your neck, torso, ankle, or anywhere in your body, depending on how you bend and twist in your daily life to balance out that pull. The primary control can easily be seen in the animal world. With a snake, you can see a very clear example of how the head leads and the body follows, propelling the snake across the ground. Or if you are riding a horse, and you pull the reins to the right, the head of the horse goes to the right, and the rest of the horse's body follows along naturally in the same direction. Another place to see the primary control clearly demonstrated is in young children. They tend to sit very upright and poised without trying. This is the primary control at work. When we as adults are conscious of the primary control, the mechanism is working well, we have balance and coordination in a coherent system, and our bodies can move with the ease and effortlessness of a child.

For most people, activating the primary control means finding our most natural and graceful state of being. For an actor, primary control is even more valuable. Primary control is an actor's touchstone—or base point—for character transformation. It is from this primary place of organization that we can transform into another character. **The primary control is a neutral starting point, sometimes called a "neutral stance."**

My experience of what many acting schools call "neutral" often manifests itself in the body as a passive deadening, the whole body becoming slightly collapsed. Actually, however, using the primary control to find a neutral starting place puts the body-mind in a very alive and dynamic state.

Exercise to Explore Primary Control

Preparation: *To begin the exercises for exploring primary control, find a comfortable stance in a room with some space around you to explore. A mirror is not necessary but may be helpful to add visual clarity.*

When you do the exercises for primary control, remember that activating primary control means activating a state of ease and natural grace. At first some of these new ideas may not feel natural. **We need to learn to distinguish between natural and habitual.** *Remember that usually what is familiar and habitual feels natural, but as your understanding grows, your idea of what is natural can change. Allow yourself to be open to these changes.*

1. *Place the tip of each index finger just inside each ear, close to the bottom of the opening. Where they would meet near the middle of your head is the top of your spine.*

This point between your ears in the center of your head is the pivotal joint where your head meets your spine: the atlanto-occipital joint. The head moves most efficiently from this point, not from the base of your neck as many people think.

Keeping your fingers in your ears, move your head upward from this central point, then forward and back, as if to lightly nod yes. Now take your fingers away. Rotate your head from this central point again forward and back, lightly lifting from that central point

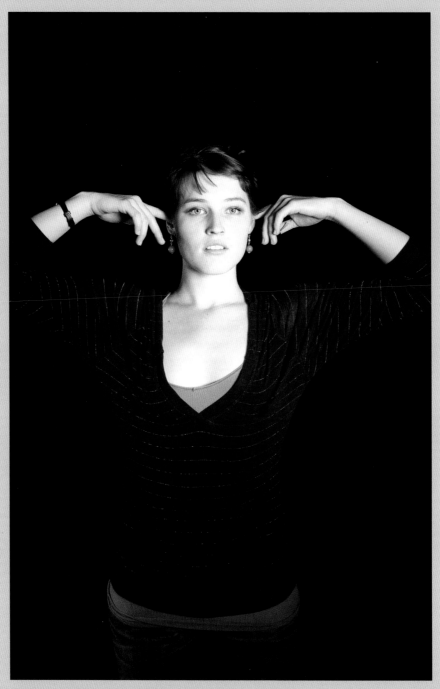

Finding the top of your spine.

between your ears where your head meets your spine. Now try rotating your head from side to side, initiating movement from that central point.

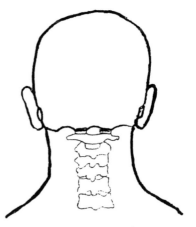

Back view of the atlanto-occipital joint.

2. *With the tips of your fingers placed again in your ears, take a walk around your space, keeping your fingers in your ears. Explore moving your head, nodding and moving it side-to-side, from the top of your spine, while walking, sitting, standing, and speaking. Allow your head always to move slightly up before each movement. This slight lift upward initiates movement. As you move around the room, ask yourself, "How does moving my head this way, slightly lifting before each movement from the top of my spine, affect the rest of my body?"*

Students often ask me, "How should I hold my head?" The real question is actually, "How is my head holding me?" The way you hold your head affects the rest of your body. If your head is dropping down onto your spine, your head is holding your spine compressed downward on the rest of your body, restricting your movement. If your head is freeing upward away from your spine, your head is allowing your whole body to release upward and move freely. Most people place their attention in their heads in order to think, but they do not often have a sense of their entire head in relationship to their body, and how it leads and directs the body to follow.

2. The Power of Habit

We all have habits, and different ways of responding to stimuli. What makes us happy? What stimulates us to feel upset? What are our habitual responses? These habits are formed by genetics, the environment, training, and many other factors and influences, including: direct experiences (good and bad), learned behavior (imitation), accidents or injuries, illnesses, emotions, chemical imbalances, trauma, stress, love, and desires. We have habitual mannerisms, like smiles or waves, and other body movements. Our habits influence the way we think, speak, breathe, and move.

As an actor, one wants to be as free and flexible as possible to transform into another person. If you are not able to recognize your own habits and mannerisms, and then to change them, your transforming possibilities remain limited. Once you begin to develop awareness of your own habits, you will open up a huge new realm of choice for yourself. Your habit will not automatically determine your response: you will then have the freedom to choose your response.

Developing awareness of habits has another important effect on a performance, in which each word, gesture, and movement of an actor tells a piece of the story to the audience. On stage you may not be aware of certain habits—raising your eyebrows, for example, clearing your throat, or leaning on one leg—but remember, everyone who watches you will see those things, even if you don't know you're doing them. The audience is not only aware of these gestures but will interpret them as significant to the story you are telling.

The work we do here is not a question of eliminating habits, but a question of reintroducing parts of the self that have, for one reason or another, become exiled. Let's say that our personality is a collection of parts, things like "The Victim," "The Golden Child," or "The Caregiver," and so on. The dominant parts are often what form your habits. There may be a "Controlling" part that likes to talk a lot and thinks it knows better than the others. A habitual pattern might develop where this part gets to speak often and in a loud voice. On the other hand, exiled parts do not get to emerge very often. Once you become aware of the dominant parts and the habits they cause, the exiled parts are set free. Then the actor has more choices and isn't beholden to the personality-driven habits. Moving forward, we won't get into the psychology of the parts, but we will deal with dominant and dormant parts of ourselves and the habits they form.

One of my students was raised in a household where her parents worked out of their house. My student loved to sing at the top of her lungs, but when her parents had clients, she needed to be quiet. Her loud singing voice went into exile, hidden away. As an actor, you can invite these parts back. That way you can have access to your full spectrum of tools as an actor. The student who had to keep her voice hidden can rediscover her strong voice, a part of herself that she kept hidden emotionally, but would come in handy if she were singing in a musical.

Exercise to Explore the Power of Habit

Preparation: *To begin the exercises to explore the power of habit, set up a chair near your phone. If you have a cell phone, have it handy.*

Before you do the exercises, take a moment and try to identify some of your own habits: of behavior, of speaking, of physicality, of thinking, and so on. Inquire into the validity of these habits in your present day life. Then think about how these habits might be able to change. Alexander said, "We can throw away the habit of a lifetime in a few minutes if we use our brain."[2]

> 1. *Pretend that the phone is ringing, then pick it up and answer. As you answer it, notice what you do with your head as you bring the phone to you. A common habit is to tilt your head toward the phone.*

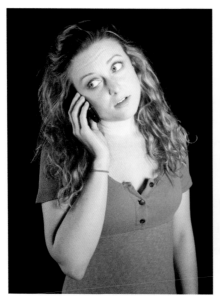 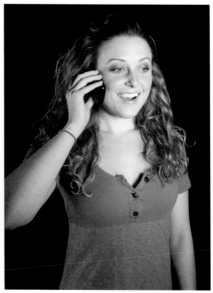

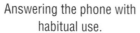

Answering the phone with habitual use. Answering the phone with improved use.

2. *Pretend the phone is ringing again, and this time, try to answer the phone without tilting your head toward the phone, or whatever other habits you may have noticed yourself doing to answer the phone in the first step of the exercise. For most people it will feel very strange to move in a way other than their habit.*

Understanding your own habits allows you to change. It might allow you to play another character that may answer the phone differently from you.

You can try this exercise with any habit. For example, most people always start walking with either their right or left leg stepping first. Try starting to walk with your nondominant leg. Or if you are sitting down, try crossing your other leg on top. If you live in the United States and have ever been to England or Australia (or vice versa), notice how difficult it is to look both ways when you cross the street, as you need to look the other way first.

You can begin to observe your own habits in daily life. Try identifying five basic actions you do during the day and your habits that might go along with those actions. When you sit down to eat, do you lean over the table? Or back away from the table? How do you get out of bed? Do you hop out? Slide? Jump out because you're running late? As you progress through to the rest of the exercises in this book, the knowledge of your own habits and mannerisms will be beneficial in helping you to use them or change them as you transform into another character.

3. Inhibition

In the Alexander Technique, the word *inhibition* has a positive meaning. In Alexander terms, inhibition means not doing the immediate response in the habitual way. **Alexander used *inhibit* as a verb:** If you inhibit the immediate response to an action or feeling, you free yourself to change your habit. Rather than saying, "I'm going to make sure my head is not moving back as I speak," you might say, "I will inhibit pulling my head back as I speak." In Alexander's case, he observed that pulling his head back and down put pressure on his larynx and constricted his voice. When we begin to observe our own use and misuse, most of us respond by wanting to fix our habitual action with a counter action. For example, "My head is pulled back. The solution is to move it forward." Let's look at why that is not the most efficient response. Alexander's head was moving back and down because he was constricting the muscles in the back of his neck. This was the first pull. If he moved his head forward to fix the position, he would be tightening the muscles in the front of his neck, and he would be adding a second pull. This would limit his freedom of motion.

Moving his head forward did not solve Alexander's problem. First, he needed to stop pulling his head back. In other words, he needed to inhibit the backward pull of his head. I often say to students, "Inhibit pulling your head back." When you release the effort of the muscles in the back of your neck and stop pulling your head back, you will feel your head move slightly forward. This is very different from pulling your head forward. The idea is not to counteract, but to release—to focus your awareness on inhibiting, or not allowing, the habitual contractive patterns of movement to take over. Often, bringing your attention to the constriction allows it to change. Recognizing, accepting, and being with your response allows it to change. *Inhibit* means (a) stopping the immediate response in order to free yourself from habitual gestures and movements, and (b) doing the same activity, but with less effort.

When you encounter a problem, most people think, "What should I do to fix it?" **The real question is, "What am I doing to cause the problem?"** Thinking about it this way allows you to discover the source of the problem, and that way you can eliminate the cause.

Give yourself some time to explore inhibition, because it is not a familiar concept in our modern fast-paced world.

Exercise to Explore Inhibition

1. *Sit at a desk or table with a pen and a piece of paper to write on. Start to write. Notice whether you are gripping the pen tightly, maybe causing your knuckles to turn a little white. If you are gripping the pen tightly, ask yourself if you can do less, hold the pen with less force. Keep asking,* **"Can I do less?" "Can I do less?"** *until you say "no."*

2. *Brushing your teeth is another example where the preparation or "set" has nothing to do with the activity. Most people grip the toothbrush like it weighs five pounds and prepare to do strenuous work with the seemingly heavy object. But the toothbrush is light, and brushing shouldn't be a strenuous activity. One only needs to hold the brush very lightly, and brush with small movements. Rather than prep for a strenuous task, what makes more sense is to take into account what*

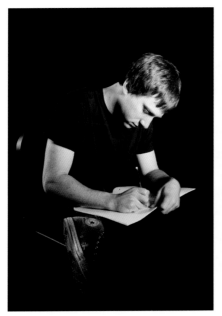 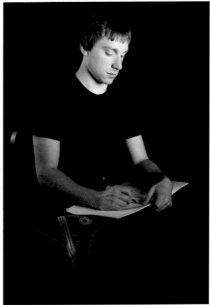

Writing with habitual tension.   Writing with "Can I do less?"

is required for the action, and respond to that. This way you meet the moment and can work clearly with what needs to be done, rather than having a disproportionate habitual response prepped before you take into account all the information of what the task actually needs.

3. *Keep exploring the concept of inhibition while trying different activities. Ask yourself: Does my preparation match the activity? Am I preparing without really being aware of the present circumstances? Can I do less, use less effort, and still accomplish the activity? Explore these principles with many activities, both on stage and off:*

   • *While speaking, does your speech speed up when you are on stage? Does your voice get higher?*

   • *When you sit down to play an instrument, do you stop breathing?*

   • *Do you use too much unnecessary effort when you walk?*

- *In your acting, can you show intense emotion using less tension in your body?*

Each of the exercises for inhibition involves recognizing what I'm calling a set. As we said, a set is a preparation to do an activity, an attitude of expectancy, that facilitates a learned response. Sets may be appropriate and suited to the activity or not. Write down your observations about how you set yourself to write, brush your teeth, walk on stage, and more, as you explored in the exercise above. For example, a set for walking onto the stage may be to hold your breath, or to brace yourself. Neither are productive. Once you observe that you have these habitual sets, and learn to inhibit them, then you are able to choose if the preparation you have been habitually doing is actually appropriate for the action.

John was having trouble playing a very powerful character. John said, "I have an idea of what powerful is, and I am setting myself up as powerful, but it just doesn't feel right." I asked him why. As he began to think about his answer, he realized, "I have so many habitual, set ideas about this character. They're really just getting in my way." John realized that his preparation was not appropriate for the action of this character. He began to inhibit some of his habitual ideas, and that created a space for new interpretations to emerge.

4. Faulty Sensory Perception

What you think that you are doing versus what you are actually doing may be two different things. Many people stand with one shoulder higher than the other, but think that their shoulders feel even, or "right." Habits that you do for a long time start to feel normal. Think about walking into a room and noticing a strange smell. After being in the room for a while, you stop noticing that there's a smell. We tend to get used to the familiar. Someone might not be able to smell their own perfume or cologne because they are so used to it, but others notice it right away.

Kinesthetic perception deals with sensations of position and movement, heaviness and lightness, holding and freeing. For example, when you stand with your arms by your sides and look straight ahead, then move your hand, you know that your hand is moving, even though you are not looking at it. This is your kinesthetic sense.

The reason you have "faulty sensory appreciation" with the kinesthetic sense is that the kinesthetic sense works partly through the spindles in the muscles. These spindles are tiny mechanisms whose function is to convey information from muscles to nerve centers in the brain about the state of the muscles, and then receive information back from the brain as to what to do about it. If a muscle is in a prolonged contracted state, the messages cannot get through to the spindles, and therefore the feedback system of the spindles does not work optimally. You cannot feel what you are doing, but you are unaware of this, because the messages are not getting from the brain to the muscles, or from the muscles to the brain. You may hold tension in your shoulders and arms that you are not aware of. If I ask you to let me hold the weight of your arm, most likely you will feel like you are letting me hold the whole weight of your arm. In reality, because of the prolonged contractive state in the muscles, you are likely still holding onto your arm and are not in fact giving me the full weight.

When you begin to change the way that you use your body, your new use may feel strange. Sometimes, when people begin to change their use, they feel pain. If you feel some pain at first, don't worry; it may be that you are feeling your habitual misuse for the first time. Now, with your increased awareness, this can change. However, if the pain persists, seek medical attention.

The exercises to explore faulty sensory perception will help you evaluate if what you are intending to do is in fact what you are actually doing.

Exercise to Explore Faulty Sensory Perception

1. *Stand in front of a mirror. Then, without looking at the mirror or your arms, reach your arms out to the sides, parallel to the floor. Then check in the mirror to see if one arm is higher than the other. Now try it with your feet. Place your feet parallel to each other without looking at them. Then look and check to see if they are actually parallel. If you tend to turn your feet out, making them parallel will feel like you are turning them in.*

2. *Many people stand with their shoulders back behind their hips, their body slightly leaning back, but they still feel straight. Stand in front of a mirror so you see yourself from a side view. Are your shoulders directly over your hips? Or are they behind your hips? If they are behind your hips, go back to your primary control and free your head away from your spine. Now let your back begin to lengthen and widen. Your shoulders will very likely now feel forward. Check your side view in the mirror to see if your shoulders are over your hips.* Students often observe themselves in disbelief when they try this exercise and see that they are not actually leaning forward.

3. *Stand facing the mirror with a chair placed behind you. As you sit in the chair, do you lift your feet or toes off the ground? Did you know that you did that, or whatever other habit you might have noticed, every time you sat down in a chair? Now try sitting down again, keeping your feet on the ground as you sit.*

I always find the concept of faulty sensory perception rather humbling. Many of us feel that we are so sure that what we feel is right, is right. But then we look in the mirror to see that we are wrong. This concept can also show up in other areas of life as well. Keep this thought in mind as you proceed through further exercises.

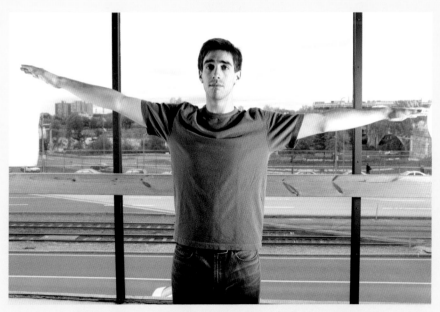

Faulty sensory perception of the arms parallel to the floor.

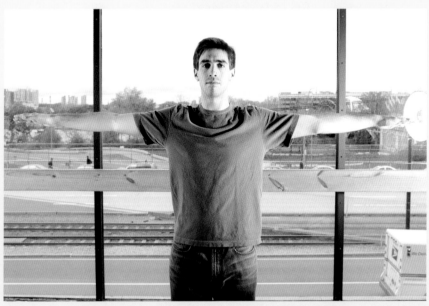

Accurate perception of the arms parallel to the floor.

5. Direction

Alexander did not believe in exercises per se. He didn't think it made sense to exercise for one hour every day, and spend the other twenty-three hours slumping down and misusing yourself. It is better to pay attention to yourself in small ways all through the day. We call this "directing."

Messages are passing all the time from the brain to the body and from the body to the brain via nerve pathways. These messages move the body, control responses, and direct the body. This is a subconscious process, even for messages sent to the voluntary muscles. To bring this process to a conscious level, Alexander devised what he called "directions." **Directions prevent faulty use and promote coordination by teaching you to think about your use at the same time that you are doing activities.**

No action is purely physical or purely mental. When you want to move your arm, you must first think that you want to move it. Directions link thought to action. A direction is a mental command. In the example of lengthening your arm, you have the intention of lengthening your arm away from your back. Then, you may feel a slight movement, a tangible reality that your arm may feel different. This is a sensorial feedback. Your arm feels longer, and has less tension. I call this "giving directions." The phrase is used a lot in talking about the Alexander work. As you read stories throughout this book that my students have shared, they will often say, "I gave my directions and then . . . happened." "When I give directions, I feel. . . ." Giving directions is a large part of my work, and key in finding a neutral place to start with your acting, or in reconnecting with your self at any point. It's a simple, effective way to check in with your mind and body, and make sure that you are not holding or constricting anywhere in your body or mind.

Directing establishes and refines connections between what you think and what you do. For example, "As I sit, I want my back to lengthen," or, "As I walk onto the stage, I don't want to stop breathing deeply." Some directions have you do something, others help you to not do something (or inhibit it), and others help prepare you for an activity.

Every thought manifests as a bodily reality. Charles Sherrington, a nineteenth-century world-renowned physiologist, said, "I may seem to stress the preoccupation of the brain with muscle. Can we stress too much that preoccupation when any path we trace in the brain leads directly or indirectly to muscle?"[3] This is an amazing fact. Most of us are not aware of this connection. This pathway allows directing to be a kind of energizing that precedes and accompanies movement.

You can learn to direct your thoughts so that you can improve yourself, rather than letting your thoughts, body, and mind work against you, which is obviously counterproductive. Directing yourself to stand up straight is not productive because it often involves bracing up. But if you direct your head to free up and away from your spine, and your back to lengthen upward and widen outward, you will stand more upright without bracing.

We can make a distinction between three types of movement: posture, muscular movement, and direction. You can see the difference between them by doing the following three exercises. Learning to give directions is a basic and essential component of the Alexander Technique. With inhibition, you learn to say "no" to what you don't want, and with direction you can say "yes" to what you do want.

Exercise to Explore Direction

This exercise simply demonstrates the concept of direction, as opposed to posture and muscular movement.

   1. Posture: hold one finger up stiffly, as if it had good posture. Notice how that feels in the rest of your body. Does your finger feel tense? Does that tension spread to the rest of your body?

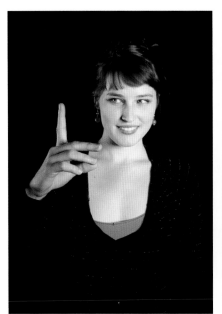 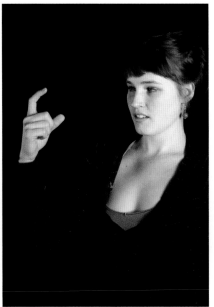

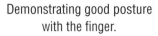

| Demonstrating good posture with the finger. | Demonstrating muscular movement with the finger. |

2. *Muscular movement: now hold your hand still and move the same finger around in space. This is an example of muscular movement. Sense how that feels different than stiffly holding your finger.*

3. *Direction: hold one finger pointing upward. Now take hold of that fingertip with your other hand and pull the finger up a bit, so it is aiming up. Then let go and keep the finger aiming up. Now the finger is not held stiffly nor being muscularly manipulated. The muscles in your finger are active, but not pushing and pulling. How does your body feel now? Is there a sense of ease and uprightness in your finger? In the rest of your body?*

This is called direction. It is not posture. It is not muscular movement. Your finger is directed. Directing the finger upward feels very different from posturing in step one, and muscularly moving the

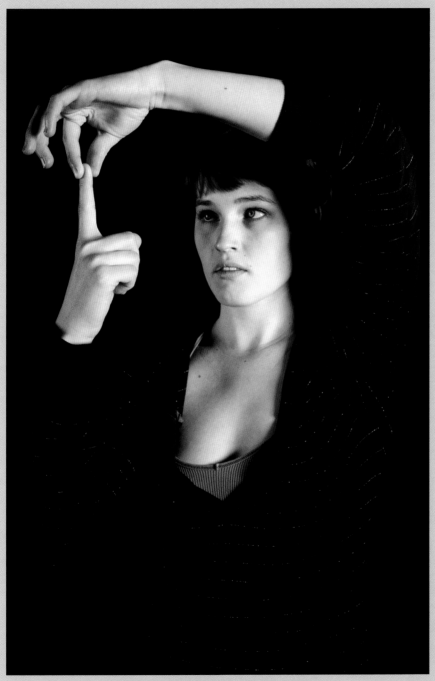

Demonstrating direction with the finger.

finger in step two. Directing your body lets it move in a helpful direction without tension. It allows your body to feel easefully upright and free.

There are directions for your whole body to improve your use. The directions are a specific set of messages that can help you recognize the small and subtle changes in your body. In the next chapter we will take a closer look at directions for the whole body, and I will define and clarify this specific process. I explain what I call "basic directions" that you will use over and over when you practice the exercises.

Although I have explained the five principles of the Alexander Technique individually, they all work together. As soon as you inhibit the shortening of your back, you direct it to lengthen. When you recognize a habit or a faulty sensory perception, you inhibit and direct. The primary control, an age-old mechanism, guides the inner organization for all the principles. These five principles allow an actor to discover his or her own resources and make choices on how to use them.

CHAPTER 5

Suspension and Support

Suspension and support are two very important concepts that determine the way we sort out balance and equilibrium. We live in a gravitational field, and therefore we are subjected to the forces of both gravity and antigravity. The force of gravity pulls us toward the earth, and the spinning of the earth creates an opposite, centrifugal force pushing outward. While gravity may give a downward, grounding pull, antigravity influences everything with an upward direction, including plants, trees, and human beings.

The intersection of these two forces creates suspension and support in the body. As you allow your neck to be free, your head frees upward so that your torso lengthens and widens. The rest of your body releases slightly downward toward the ground. The ground then supports you, and that support carries up through your legs, your spine, and your head. The forces of gravity and antigravity act on your body to create suspension from the top of your head, and support moving through your feet from the ground. Any real concept of up has a concept of down that goes along with it, and conversely any real down also has an up.

This phenomenon can also be explained by saying that there is a mutual attraction between the earth and any object sitting on it. As much weight or mass as I put down into the earth, the earth matches that mass with an upward force. For example, you might not feel like you weigh the amount of pounds you would see if you stepped on a scale. The analogy is easy to see if we use water, another surface on the earth, instead of land. Picture a boat floating on the water. The boat is supported by the exact amount of force that it exerts on the water. Thus we say it is floating. Given this analogy, it is interesting to note that one of the common phrases spoken after an Alexander session is, "I feel like I'm floating." Perhaps the following explorations will allow you to feel this.

Suspension

Many systems of movement training talk about alignment and stacking the building blocks of the body one on top of another. This way of thinking implies that the body is a compression system, in which the parts stack up for balance. But when you look at a skeleton, you see this is not the case, because you cannot stack your bones to balance them. There are no horizontal surfaces for bones

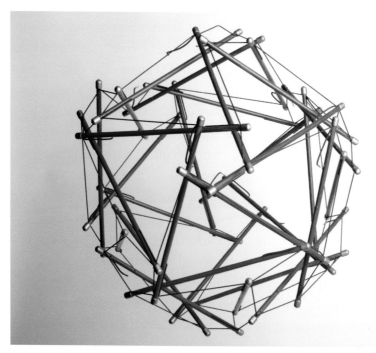

A tensegrity structure.

to rest on. The body is a suspension system, which means that all the muscles are slightly extended or lengthened for balance and efficient functioning. **Our system is more a tensegrity structure.** The American engineer Buckminster Fuller, who designed the geodesic dome, coined the word *tensegrity*. It means a combination of tension and integrity, and it demonstrates suspension. In the image, the wooden sticks, which can be likened to the bones of the body, get their shape from the elastics, which function similarly to muscles. In the tensegrity, the elastics are all slightly expanded while holding the sticks together. **The web of suspension creates an expanded container.** This expansion allows buoyancy, lightness, and a tensional balance. It works the same way in the body—this expansion allows for freedom of movement, breath, and thought.

Exercise to Explore Suspension

Preparation: *Prepare for this exercise by simply standing in a cleared space, and thinking about the idea of tensegrity and expansion.*

I call this an exercise, but it is not about gross motor movements. Read the directions and allow yourself to respond with small changes, micromovements. There's no need to make any large manipulations. Learn to recognize and appreciate the small and subtle changes that take place in your body.

1. *Beginning with your head: Sense the top of your spine where the top of your spine meets your head, between your ears. As you sense the top of your spine, allow your whole head, including the back of your head, to free a touch forward, and slightly upward.* **Note that your neck does not go forward.** *The forward and up of your head is really your head not dropping back and down.*

2. *As you observe your head freeing slightly forward and up, away from your back, your back can then open, or lengthen and widen a bit.*

Most people mistakenly think of their back as spanning from the base of the neck to the waist. However, functionally, your spine actually goes from the middle of your ears, as we explored earlier by putting your finger in your ear to find the top of your spine, all the way down to your hip sockets, where your leg bends. Be sure your back lengthens all the way down to your hip sockets, so that your hip sockets can be free. In my exercises, your back also includes the front of your body, or your whole torso. Thus lengthening and widening your back can provide space for your internal organs and for your nervous system.

> 3. *Now bring your attention to your shoulders. Try not to pull your shoulders forward or back, or up or down. You want to allow your shoulders to free out to the sides, or widen. This widening continues out to your arms.*

The old "pull your shoulders back" may appear to work on the surface, but this method is really just pulling backward on the already present pull forward. It is true that your shoulders want to sit on your back and slightly down, but that only works efficiently if you have widened your shoulders out to the sides first, making room for them to settle more toward the back.

> 4. *Now notice your ribs. Ribs attach onto your sternum with cartilage (flexible connective tissue) enabling them to move. Your ribs attach with moveable joints to your spine in back, also encouraging movement to take place, especially as you breathe. As you breathe in and out, allow your ribs to move with your breath, moving on your sternum in the front, and your spine in the back.*
> 5. *Now think about your knees. Knees bend forward. They do not bend back. Knees going backward, or locking your knees back, is called hyperextension. It is a very common habit. Try to be aware of your knees as you stand, and make sure you are*

not locking them backward. Then, as you bend, let your knees
go straight forward, out over your toes. This way the knees
won't want to bow out or aim inward, as in knock-knees.

6. *Now pay attention to your ankles. Your ankles want to be*
free and not held, especially the front of your ankles. Make
sure you are not holding tension in the front of your ankles.

If you tend to lean forward, your ankles have to grab and tighten
in order to keep you from falling over. Make sure that the tendon
that connects the top of the front of your foot to the bottom of the
front of your leg is not popping out. If it is popping out, it means
that the tendon is overworking. In the early days of ballet, dancers
wore ballet slippers that had ribbons that crossed in front of that
tendon, which was meant to keep the tendon from popping out and
prevent injury.

7. *Bring your awareness to your heels. There is a spot one inch*
in from the back of your heel. As you stand, allow this spot
to feel its contact with the ground. The rest of your foot then
spreads forward, like the webbing on a duck's foot. As your
foot spreads, or widens, this engages the reflexes on the bot-
tom of your foot to take you upright. You want to have even
contact from front to back on each foot, and you want to
have balance from side to side on each foot.

8. *As you feel the overall sensation of suspension from your*
head down through to your heels, let your body imbibe this
expansive state. Do you feel the floating sensation?

As they explored suspension, actors have found: "My breath
flows like never before." "The room is brighter." "I'm finally
connected to my voice." "My thinking is so much clearer." "I'm
awake." These statements all emerge from an opening into an
expanded self. This expansion includes your whole body. As you
experience your body slightly expanded in all directions, this is the

feeling of suspension. As the expansion hits the ground, this leads us to support.

Support

Support is an important element on many levels. If you don't understand that you are supported, you will try to hold yourself up, often with your shoulders. But if you understand that you are a whole being, and on the ground already—meaning that you will not fall down because you are already supported by the ground—then there is no need to hold yourself up.

When you have some sense of being supported, you often experience a feeling of lightness. It is not that you have lost weight in these few moments. What happens is that we tend to exert force to make ourselves heavier. We weight ourselves and pull ourselves downward, off our support, with muscular energy, and blame gravity for

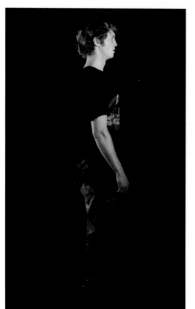

Standing with suspension and support.

it. Gravitational forces actually give us our uprightness. If you have ever seen a photo of an astronaut in space, their shoulders are often hunched over, and they do not have the uprightness that the gravitational forces give us on earth. When we stop pulling ourselves downward, we feel lighter. This is called **kinesthetic lightness.**

One of my students once said, "I felt a lightness in my body that I've been waiting for my whole life, really without even being aware of it." This is an example of feeling that kinesthetic lightness, the support from the ground, leading to a natural uprightness that is not stiff or held. When you are standing with this kinesthetic lightness, all your muscles are slightly expanded, creating equilibrium. When you stand off this balance, your system has to contract somewhere to keep you from falling.

Exercise to Explore Support

Preparation: *Find a comfortable place to stand. Again, I call this an exercise, but it is not about gross motor movements. Read the directions, and allow yourself to respond with small changes.*

1. *Bring your awareness to the bottoms of your feet.*
2. *Let the bottoms of your feet feel the floor. Notice how and where they meet the floor. Some parts have contact with the floor, and others are often pulling up off the floor. Just notice; don't try to fix anything.*
3. *Now become aware that the ground is under you, and allow the floor to support you. Notice how the rest of your body responds to the support.*
4. *Let the support come up through your body.*
5. *Let your ankles be free enough to receive that support from the ground.*
6. *Let your knees be free enough to let the support come through.*
7. *Let your hip sockets be less held, so that the support can come up through, and to lengthen up your whole back, and spread out to your arms.*
8. *Let your head free upward from the ground.*

This exercise allows you to feel the support of the ground, all the way up through the top of your head and neck. Notice what it is like to feel your feet supported by the ground in this way. Can you feel that there is less need to "hold" yourself up? Do you feel lighter from the support? The result of being supported is less muscle tension, and less pulling down. Learn to use the support of the ground. It is always there and available for you.

Many people talk about "grounding," and "ground" themselves by pushing their body weight into the ground, trying to feel planted there. But this method of pushing weight down is almost more like "grinding" into the ground, rather than grounding. **When I**

say, "Allow the ground to support you," I mean to have a sense
of your feet in contact with the ground, and then use that contact
to come up, not to go down. This way, your body weight is not
dropped downward toward the ground, but conversely is lifted
upward. It may feel counterintuitive that your upper body goes
up and your heels drop down, but letting your feet drop down to
accept the support of the ground is what gives you the base for
the lift upward. Another way to think about it is to have a slight
push into the floor, or to oppose the floor, which also allows you
to come more upright.

> 9. *When you have even contact with the floor with the front
> and back of your foot, you can receive maximum support.
> Repeat the support exercise with this awareness and allow
> that contact to bring you upward.*

The support exercise is an invaluable tool for an actor. It can
bring you back to your awareness of yourself to inhabit your body
and feel your inherent strength. As you are connected to yourself,
you can make choices about how you move and think. We all feel
more secure when we are supported.

After doing the support exercise, one student said, "I found
it to be nothing less than life-changing because I began to truly
understand the meaning of support, being totally supported by the
ground. The ground felt alive. My feet were having a conversation
with the ground. This newfound understanding of the basic concept opened up many doors for me in my work. I began to gain an
incredibly heightened sense of awareness that I had never experienced before. I'm able to give and receive more as I'm acting." Isn't
that what acting is all about—being able to listen to your fellow
actors and being comfortable enough in your own skin to be able
to respond in the moment?

When you have suspension and support, there is no sense of
effort in standing or moving. When you go off your support, or

SUSPENSION AND SUPPORT

slacken or overtense your suspension, your system responds with a contracting effort to hold you up and keep you from falling. This contracting interferes with other activities like speaking or breathing. When you move into an activity like walking, this contraction is perceived as effort. The effort you feel is equal to the amount you are pulling yourself off balance or working against yourself. You must discover what your character's support and suspension are after you have sorted out your own.

When you embody suspension and support, you can feel your full stature. Your full stature is you as full and expanded as you can be. This is not a rigid or puffed-up stance, but your body will feel slightly expanded and toned. When you embody suspension and support, your full stature includes everything that you are, not more and not less. Full stature often includes a feeling of self-confidence, because you are aware and engaging your whole sense of self, not ignoring or hiding anything.

The combination of suspension and support is a model for healthy functioning in the body. It provides an overall energized starting place for the body. The basic directions below combine the principles of suspension and support to provide you with a set of simple phrases that guide you to this organization.

Basic Directions

Giving basic directions is a fundamental component of my work. As we learned earlier, directions are the connector between thought and action. They are a way to move the body to function in its optimal form, without excess muscular tension. The basic directions provide a simple set of instructions that gently allows the body to find its optimal setting, in tandem with the concepts of suspension and support that we just explored.

~ 53 ~

Giving Basic Directions

Preparation: *You can do these basic directions sitting, standing, or lying down with your knees up, feet resting flat on the floor. Repeat the phrases to yourself, giving yourself a few moments to feel what happens in your body as you allow it to respond.*

Begin with suspension:

- *Bring my attention to the top of my spine.*
- *Allow my neck to be free.*
- *Allow my head to free forward and up, or away from my spine.*
- *Allow my back to lengthen and widen.*
- *Allow my shoulders to widen out of my back, my elbows to free away from my shoulders, and my wrists to free away from my elbows.*
- *Allow my ribs to move with my breath on my sternum and spine.*
- *Allow my knees to release slightly forward and away, and not to lock.*
- *Allow my feet to be on the ground.*
- *Allow the ground to support me.*
- *Allow my ankles, knees, and hips to be open to receive the support.*
- *Allow the support from the ground to come up through my legs, spine, arms, and head.*
- *Allow myself to breathe and to notice the room.*

Or begin with support:

- *Allow my feet to be on the ground.*
- *Allow the ground to support me.*
- *Allow my ankles, knees, and hips to be open to receive the support.*

- *Allow the support from the ground to come up through my legs, spine, arms, and head.*
- *Allow myself to breathe, and notice the room.*
- *Allow my neck to be free.*
- *Allow my head to free forward and up, or away from my spine.*
- *Allow my back to lengthen and widen.*
- *Allow my shoulders to widen out of my back, my elbows to free away from my shoulders, and my wrists to free away from my elbows.*
- *Allow my ribs to move with my breath on my sternum and spine as I notice the room.*

Various versions of these basic directions are repeated throughout this book. They set a template to move from, a way of getting your body-mind to an energized neutral state. This is what I call "giving directions." These directions precede and accompany many of the exercises. Become familiar with these basic directions, and explore them doing various activities. You may even want to memorize them. What they mean to you might change as you work through the book, as your use begins to change.

Working with giving basic directions, students have shared things like: "As I give my basic directions I feel like I'm living in a different place than I lived before." "I feel like a coiled spring ready for action." "I feel a new way of making contact with the world." "I feel more confident in myself."

Basic directions are a very powerful tool. They can help you breathe more fully, and reduce pressure on your joints to alleviate bodily aches and pains. They also help you to become more aware of the world around you.

Using the basic directions can be very helpful in your acting in many ways. You can do them in rehearsal, before a performance, or even during one. A student of mine talked about his experience

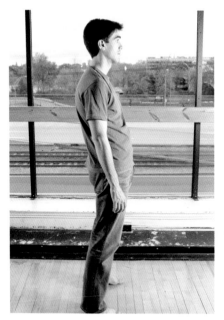 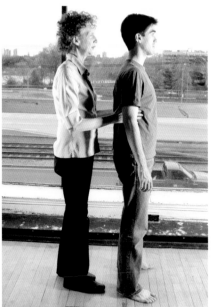

Standing without basic directions.   Standing with basic directions.

of giving basic directions while working on a play: "I was waiting backstage for an entrance when I was seized with a feeling of
anxiety and stress that I could not get rid of. Rather than denying
this fact and trying to bypass it, I went through my basic directions, found the ground, and allowed the feeling to exist. I'll be
dammed if that feeling didn't just go away during the scene. This
work allows me to be present with whatever is going on." The
basic directions helped the student to stop the worry and anxiety
and reconnect with himself in the present moment, which made
his fear melt away.

CHAPTER 6

Breathing

Notice your breathing pattern now. How do you use yourself to breathe? Are your breaths short and quick? Long and slow? Do you pause between breaths? Do you feel like you can never quite get enough air? If you are anxious or trying too hard to do something, chances are that your breath is limited. If you are comfortable and unstressed, chances are your breath is flowing.

The importance of breathing cannot be over emphasized. Breathing is not only about oxygen coming in and carbon dioxide going out; breathing is also your connection to life and to the life force that sustains you. The place where you meet your life force is very special, even sacred. When your breath comes in, you get a spark of life and you absorb as much of this life force as you can.

Unfortunately, for most people the amount of air absorbed is rather limited. The vital lung capacity, the amount of air your lungs can hold, is rarely at its maximum. Because there are various blocks, the breath does not go in and out freely. All of this creates your own unique breathing patterns.

Your breathing is your inspiration and your expiration. Your breath inspires you with creativity, life force, and oxygen. Oxygen is said to elevate spirits and stimulate activity. Your expiration, the process of breathing out, removes carbon dioxide from your body. Carbon dioxide is said to have a stressful and depressing effect on the body.

How you breathe cannot be separated from how you use yourself. If you are collapsed and pulling downward for one reason or another, it is hard to have room to breathe well. As you pay attention to and improve your use, your breathing will improve. The following explanations and exercises will help lead you in this direction.

Breath denotes character. Your breath shows what you are thinking, feeling, sensing, imagining, and dreaming. It reflects your emotional life and underpins your behavior. Your past history determines your specific breathing pattern. Your biography becomes your biology. Your body tells the whole story. In other words, the events that happen in your life become part of your bodily systems, including the circulatory, respiratory, and nervous systems affecting your cells, muscles, and organs. If your life story includes growing up in an unsafe environment, it is likely that your respiratory system has been compromised. Your quality and quantity of breath tend to be habitual and keep you locked in certain habits and patterns.

One common habit is holding your breath to prevent yourself from feeling certain feelings. For actors, this limits your transformability, and you would be wise to change. You want to be able to feel the feelings of the various characters that you play. To effectively change this habit of holding your breath, first you need the physiological knowledge and understanding of how the breath works. Second, you need to see your own unique patterns of breathing related to your emotional makeup and feelings. You will see how your breathing patterns connect to your overall human experience. You need to know your own tendencies in order to change them to fully embody another character.

Breathing is not an activity. It is a response to activity. Breathing is not something that you "do," like speaking or singing, but it is a built-in, automatically regulated function. When you walk, you breathe. When you run, you breathe faster, without you needing to "do" anything. The same is true with your voice. If you need to speak louder or stronger, you use your breath in a different way to get more vocal power and resonance. It is not something that you consciously do.

To begin to understand and investigate your own breath, start by asking these questions. "Am I breathing fully or minimally?" "Do I feel deep, full, satisfying breaths or shallow, unfulfilling breaths?" "If I hold my breath, I interfere with the normal breathing cycle. What does that do to the rest of my body?" "How much do my ribs and belly move?" "How long are my inhale and exhale?" "How often do I yawn because my body needs oxygen?" (Yawning is a sign of needing oxygen.) "How heavy or light does my chest feel?" "How much do I collapse down or aim up on my exhale?" "As I speak, what happens to my breath? Does my belly tighten?"

You must know all of these details about your own breath before you can take on another person's breath. How you breathe will make the audience believe or not believe that you are living in the imaginary circumstances of a play.

Three-Dimensional Breathing

There are many opinions on how and where to breathe. Some teachers say you should breathe into your belly. Some say breathe into your back. Some say move your ribs. Others say don't move your ribs. Many say do something called diaphragmatic breathing. But what exactly is that? I have heard many varying answers as to what diaphragmatic breathing is from different sources. A combination of what I call three-dimensional breathing and optimal breathing uses the diaphragm in a way that might be described as diaphragmatic breathing. First, we will take a closer look at three-dimensional breathing.

I believe that breathing is a three-dimensional activity in the torso, and that it radiates out to the arms, legs, and head. The "how" of breathing has a very specific coordination that will continue to be described, demonstrated, and experienced in this chapter. The "where" to breath will become clear when you understand the anatomical makeup of the respiratory system. The ribs attach in front to the sternum with cartilage. Cartilage is very movable, like the tip of your nose. The ribs attach in back to your spine with moveable joints above and below the ribs. Both front and back attachments of the ribs are designed for motion. This implies that the ribs are supposed to move as you breathe. Begin to explore this idea by using the following exercise.

Exercise to Explore Three-Dimensional Breathing

Preparation: *Stand or sit comfortably.*

1. *Three-dimensional breath has a side-to-side quality to it, because the ribs attach to the sternum in front and the spine in back. As the lungs fill with air, the ribs open to the sides. Put your hands on the sides of your ribs and feel your ribs and torso moving sideways as you breathe. Then remove your hands and sense the movement.*

2. *Three-dimensional breath has an up-and-down quality to it because the diaphragm travels up and down. Put one hand on top of your torso by your collarbone, and the other at the bottom, on your belly. Feel your ribs and torso moving up and down. Now take your hands off and just sense the movement. Your lungs fill from bottom to top as you breathe, and the top of your lungs is one inch above each collarbone. Be sure to fill this top section with breath.*

3. *Three-dimensional breath has a front-to-back quality to it because of the expansion of the lungs. Put one hand on the front of your torso on your sternum, and the other on your back. Feel your ribs and torso moving front to back as you breathe.* **Because the bulk of the tissue of your lungs is in back, you want to make sure you feel your back moving.** *(You may have noticed that when a doctor checks your lungs, she always puts the stethoscope on your back first to feel the movement of your lungs.) Now take your hands off and sense the movement.*

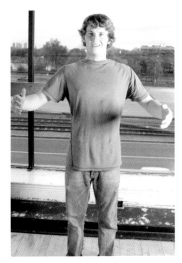
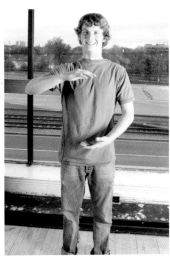
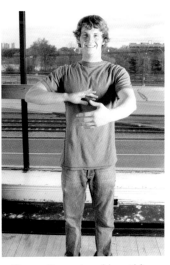

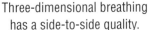

| Three-dimensional breathing has a side-to-side quality. | Three-dimensional breathing has an up-and-down quality. | Three-dimensional breathing has a front-to-back quality. |

After exploring this exercise, do you have a greater sense of your breath? Did some of the movement surprise you? Since many people use very little of their breathing capacity, this exercise can be very eye-opening in how much breath we can actually circulate in and out.

A student who I'll call Sandra came in for a lesson. She was having trouble taking a deep breath, because she said one of her ribs hurt. She was concerned about her ability to move around in rehearsal because of this pain in her chest. Sandra had had a bad cough a few weeks before and had coughed so much that her rib still hurt now even though the cough was gone. She thought perhaps her rib was fractured or dislocated. I looked at the way she was standing. Her upper back was leaning way back, and her bottom front ribs were jutting forward so that her ribs were not moving freely on her sternum or spine. She was not able to get a three-dimensional breath. I pointed this out to her and helped her shift her back and rib cage so that she could also feel her breath in her back. She could then take a deep breath with no pain, and sighed a sigh of relief.

Her next rehearsal was "a joy," she said. It's not that Sandra's rib was actually injured, but the way her body was leaning on her ribs was causing her pain. Once we reorganized the way she was holding her back and ribs, she was able to breathe fully and optimally, allowing for three-dimensional breath and for her pain to go away.

Optimal Breath

A healthy physical body has a springlike quality, a bounce in the step, a fluidity to movement. **An optimal, healthy breath also has that springlike quality.** As you learn to connect your conscious awareness to your breath, which is part of your life force, you will find your breathing can have this springlike quality. There is a freedom to the movement of the breath in and out and the ribs expanding and contracting. This is also called a reflex inhale, which means that you do not need to do something, like suck air in, to take a breath. An optimal breath also includes movement of the whole torso, and three-dimensional breathing, especially engaging the ribs and belly.

Most people choose one of two major tendencies for breathing. One is to collapse both the spine and the ribs to exhale. This is often called "relaxing." The other is to hold up and tense both the spine and upper chest. This is often called "good posture." Neither of these habits foster the natural springlike quality in the breath. The springlike quality is an important aspect in the entire system, as it keeps things moving reflexively. Think of the obvious bouncing quality in a trampoline. You jump down on it and it springs back up. In a similar way, **the ribs in the rib cage are structurally spring-loaded.** Each rib is individually spring-loaded along the sternum and spine. If a rib were to split in half, each side would spring open toward the sternum or spine. When you exhale properly, all of your ribs spring back open to inhale, making space for a new breath. This can make you feel alive and energetic. To foster this springlike quality, allow your spine to lengthen upward, while your ribs drape downward as you are letting the air out. This is a very beautiful dynamic, the spine going up and the ribs going down as you exhale. Then your ribs swing open to inhale.

This dynamic can happen because of the manubrium. The manubrium is a small bone at the top of your sternum. Where the manubrium meets the sternum is a cartilage joint that is made for flexibility. Because of this flexibility, your collarbone and upper torso can stabilize upward while your ribs drape downward to remove the air from your lungs as you exhale.

It is the importance of the exhale that is to be noted here. Many people incorrectly think that the inhale is the important phase in the act of breathing, and they try to control it. People say, "Take a breath" (or "tank up" when singing). This controlled taking of breath places unhealthy pressure on the diaphragm, because it tenses muscles in the neck and chest that do not need to be involved in breathing.

Because most people are busy taking a breath, they do not pay much attention to the process of exhaling. This is not a good plan. If you have not exhaled completely, carbon dioxide is left in the lungs. The system detects this, and sees that there is too much carbon dioxide and not enough oxygen; it does the only thing it knows how to do: ask for more oxygen, causing an inhale. Since the lungs are still partially filled with carbon dioxide, not as much oxygen can get in. A vicious cycle is set in motion. You keep inhaling to get more oxygen, but the oxygen cannot get into the lungs because they are already filled with carbon dioxide, which then causes you to keep trying to inhale for more oxygen. This habit can lead to respiratory weakness and illness because it weakens the system with a buildup of carbon dioxide.

However, when you exhale completely, your body is designed to take a reflex inhale. By getting all the air out of your lungs, you create a partial vacuum, and the air comes in as a reflex. This is what

I call an optimal breath. Optimal breath means you do not suck air in to "take" a breath, but allow the breath to come in as a reaction to the springlike motion of the ribs, allowing the lungs to effortlessly fill with oxygen, and easily exhale the carbon dioxide.

Detailed Explanation of an Optimal Breath and a Reflex Inhale

Below is a step-by-step outline of how the optimal breath works. I begin with the exhale because that is the most misunderstood phase of the cycle.

- *Exhale: as you breath out, the diaphragm rises and domes up under the ribs and pushes air out of the lungs, and your belly goes in toward your spine.*
- *Inhale: as the lungs fill with air from bottom to top, the dome-shaped diaphragm flattens as it descends for an inhale. As the diaphragm goes down, it displaces the viscera (the internal organs) in your belly area, and your belly expands out.*
- *Exhale: the ribs fold around the diaphragm as it rises within the rib cage and moves air out of the lungs. Muscles, both voluntary and involuntary, function synergistically to produce a greater flow of air out of the lungs. The stronger the diaphragm is, the higher it rises, giving you a minimum residual volume of carbon dioxide stored in the lungs at the end of the exhale.*
- *Inhale: now that the diaphragm is rising and falling smoothly, the ribs expanding and contracting accordingly, the inhale that follows becomes a neurological response, or reflex inhale.*

I suggest that you take time here to familiarize yourself with the details of an optimal breath before you begin the next exercise. My teaching experience has shown me that many people do not understand the reflex inhale clearly.

Exercise to Explore Optimal Breath with a Reflex Inhale

An optimal breath produces simple and effective breathing to strengthen and redevelop the diaphragm, an involuntary muscle. Breathing involves both voluntary and involuntary muscles. This exercise helps you sort out when to inhibit the voluntary muscles in order to allow the involuntary muscles to work.

Preparation: *As you begin to do the following breathing exercises, lie on your back, your head on a one- or two-inch book, with your knees bent, and your feet flat. If you have no book, your head will very likely be pulled back and down, because it will fall too far below the line of your spine resting on the ground. This is why it is helpful to place a small item under your head. If a book is too hard for you, you can use a folded towel. Moving forward, I'll give the instruction to "prepare for lying-down work," meaning getting into this lying-down position with a book or towel supporting your head and your knees bent up with your feet flat on the floor.*

For the breathing exercises, prepare for lying-down work. You can also let your legs lie straight and place a cushion under your knees. Let yourself settle into the floor or mat, and let whatever is under you support you.

1. *Begin by observing your breath. Feel it flowing in and out. What do you notice? Does your breath feel full? Shallow? Fast? Slow? Is there movement in your torso? If so, where?*
2. *As you exhale, allow the exhale to be complete, letting all the air flow out from your lungs. Do not cut it short.* **Extend the exhale, taking it to its complete conclusion.**
3. *As you inhale, allow the air to come in, or drop in. Place your hands on your belly and then on your ribs to feel the movement. It can sometimes feel like the breath is "swooping" in.*

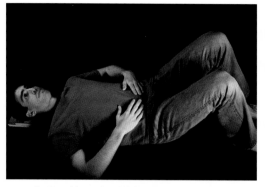

Optimal breath with hands on the belly.

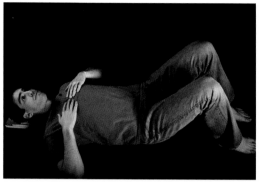

Optimal breath with hands on the chest.

4. *As you extend your exhale again, do not force, squeeze, or push the air out. As you exhale, think of the air going up along your spine as you lengthen your spine. Allow your ribs to move on your sternum in front and on your spine in back. Feel your back moving.*

5. *As you inhale, don't suck or pull the air in, and don't lift your shoulders.*

6. *As you exhale, the diaphragm rises and the belly drops toward the floor.*

7. *As you inhale, the diaphragm drops down and flattens or spreads out, and your belly expands.*

8. *After you have become familiar with an optimal breath lying down, roll over onto your side, and stand up. Now stand and practice an optimal breath. As you exhale, your ribs drape down as your spine aims up. The line of energy of your draping ribs extends down through your feet (heels, toes, and arches) to the floor. It feels as if your ribs drop to the floor and bounce back up. This is the element of the springlike quality that enlivens your whole system, body, mind, and self, as you stand and move through life.*

An optimal breath with a reflex inhale both calms and energizes you at the same time. Once you stop holding the muscles in your ribs and your belly that are interfering with your breathing mechanisms, there is greater airflow and larger vital lung capacity. You are able to process more oxygen, making you feel more energized, as your life force is moving through you. As you breathe more comfortably, it also may help you feel calm and centered. This is good preparation for both daily life and performance.

Inefficient Breathing Patterns to Watch For

People develop many inefficient breathing patterns. Three of the most common are paradoxical or backward breathing, accessory breathing, and belly breathing. As an actor, noting these inefficient breathing patterns has two benefits: you can improve your own breathing, and you can use the inefficient patterns to convey specific character traits. If you take a moment to practice these three inefficient breathing patterns, you will begin to learn to recognize the patterns in your own breathing.

1. Paradoxical breathing or backward breathing: on the inhale, the belly goes in, and on the exhale, and belly goes out, rather than the other way around.
2. Accessory breathing: using extra, or accessory, muscles for the breathing process. It usually includes some form of lifting the shoulders and using the muscles of the upper chest and neck in order to empty and fill the lungs.
3. Belly breathing: breathing only into your belly with no rib movement. This usually involves a downward collapse of the ribs, chest, and upper body. Your lungs fill with air, not your belly. Your belly responds.

Can you notice that each of these patterns creates a different internal state in your body or your emotions? Can you feel the difference between an optimal breath and the inefficient breathing patterns?

Extending the Exhale

As we've seen, most people have an excursion of their diaphragm that is less than optimal, meaning that their diaphragm is not as strong as it could be and they don't fully expel carbon dioxide from their lungs. Maximum motion of the diaphragm is four and a half inches, but most people have less than one and a half inches of motion, using only a third of their capacity. This shows that the diaphragm is in a weakened state. As you learn to extend your exhale, you can strengthen your diaphragm.

Exercise to Explore Extending the Exhale: Silent "La La La"

As you continue to extend your exhale, you strengthen your diaphragm even more, as it lowers on the inhale and rises on the exhale. A strengthened diaphragm will help in easing the natural flow of your breath in and out.

Preparation: *This exercise can be done sitting, standing, walking, or lying down.*

1. *Do a few cycles of optimal breathing, paying attention to your exhale. Is it cut short? Is it forced?*
2. *Now say "la la la" silently as you breathe out. To do this, your tongue moves from behind your top teeth to behind your bottom teeth. It does not involve your jaw; don't move your jaw up and down while doing the silent "la la la." Continue the "la la la" for the entire exhale.*

The silent "la la la" tricks the glottis into staying open longer and extends the exhale without pressure. By extending the exhale as far as possible, it triggers a reflex inhale. This way you don't "take" a breath, but the breath springs in without muscular effort. Constant, undemanding use of the diaphragm—which has become

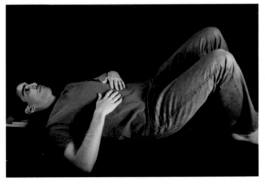
Breathing with extended exhale.

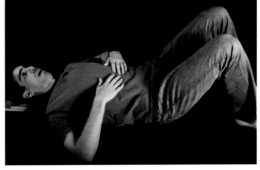
Breathing with silent "la la la."

a weakened muscle in most people due to misuse, underuse, or improper use—enables the diaphragm to develop.

One acting student I worked with was having an asthma attack and ran to her apartment to get her inhaler and medicine. As she got to the door, she realized that she had forgotten her keys. Becoming aware that she was locked out of her apartment, her breathing became more labored and she began to get frightened, both for her own health and about performing in her show that night. Then, as she tells the story, "I figured, 'What the hell. I'll try some of the breathing exercises from Betsy's class.'" She lay down on the floor in the hallway of her apartment and repeated silent "la la las" as she extended her exhale. After doing this for a few rounds, she was able to keep her asthma attack at a manageable level until her landlord came with the keys to let her in. And she was able to go on stage that night with no breathing problems whatsoever.

Breath and Sound

As you practice, the silent "la la la" will begin to strengthen your diaphragm. The next thing you want to add to continue to strengthen and redevelop your diaphragm is sound. When you are just breathing, there is space between the vocal folds. The vocal folds produce sound when they touch and vibrate together. Adding the resistance of the vocal folds as you breathe out strengthens the diaphragm, as it has more to push against. This is like a weight lifter adding weights to build strength.

Exercise to Explore Breath and Sound: Counting Exercise

Preparation: *Lie on your back, your head on a book, with your knees bent and feet flat, or let your legs straighten with a cushion under your knees. Let yourself settle into the floor or mat, and let whatever is under you support you.*

1. *Do one exhale of silent "la la la" so the inhale comes as a reflex.*
2. *Count "1, 2, 3, 4, 5" out loud on the exhale. Then do a silent "la la la" to finish whatever breath you have to complete the exhale.*
3. *Inhale again, this time counting "1, 2, 3, 4, 5, 6, 7, 8, 9, 10" on the exhale. Do a silent "la la la" to finish the exhale.*
4. *Inhale, counting "1, 2, 3, 4, 5, 6, 7, 8, 9, 10, 1, 2, 3, 4, 5" on the exhale. Do silent "la la la" to finish the exhale.*
5. *Keep increasing the count by five, but never count beyond the number ten. Remember to lengthen and widen your back while you exhale.*
6. *As you repeat more sets of one-to-ten counts, try saying them in a singsongy manner, using different pitches, so that the diaphragm is still rising and moving smoothly. If you say the numbers in a staccato fashion, the diaphragm will be moving in a jerky fashion.*
7. *Only grow the count as high as you can go without tensing your belly and without pulling your shoulders together to squeeze the exhale out. Allow your shoulders to widen as your torso is lengthening.*

8. *Stop if you feel yourself overly tensing and start the process again, from the last number set you felt completely at ease with (perhaps four sets of tens). Don't push yourself to go farther than you're comfortable with. But as you practice this exercise, you will find yourself being able to count more and more sets of ten.*

It is important to link the breath work with the Alexander work. In both teachings we see that **the exhale is the activity that requires more attention than the inhale.** As you lengthen and widen your torso for a complete exhale, you are able to get the reflex inhale, which also includes a lengthening and widening of your torso.

After doing work on extending the exhale, a student I taught spoke about a character who was very sexually powerful that she was having trouble fully connecting with. "I could not seem to get out of my head and into my lower body," she said. "But last night I did the Counting Exercise before I went on stage, and I had tremendous power in my sexuality, and my lower body in general." The Counting Exercise helped the student deepen and expand her breathing, giving her a wider range of feeling and connection to her body, and enabling her to be more in tune with her character.

Breath and Movement

As we saw earlier, breath is not an activity. It is a response to activity, and it accompanies your thoughts; your breath responds to what is going on in your system. You want to learn to pay attention to your breathing as you respond to your environment. You want to be able to move, to be active, and to be with other people and still breathe fully.

Exercise to Explore Breath and Movement

You can do this exercise by yourself, with a partner, or with a group.

Preparation: *Stand in a comfortable space.*

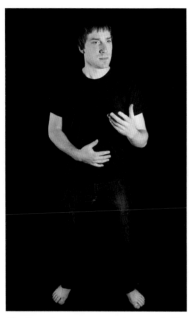

Feeling the movement in your belly as you stand and breathe.

1. *As you stand, breathe with your hands on your belly to feel the movement. Can you stand and continue breathing? It sounds like an odd question, but often outside interests stop your breath. As soon as you think of a thought about the future or past, your breath is responding to that new thought and not to feeling your belly in the present moment.*

2. *Give basic directions: allow your neck to be free so that your head can free forward and up, and allow your torso to lengthen and widen.*

3. *Repeat the silent "la, la, la" as you exhale, to slightly extend your exhale.*

4. *Allow your ribs to move without your spine collapsing.*

5. *Breathe with your hands on your chest to feel the movement. Do not force or manipulate your breath.*

6. *Allow the air to come in and go out. Let the breath drop in.*

7. *Notice the three-dimensional quality of the breath as your whole back, torso, and ribs expand and contract.*

8. *Notice how your breath relates to your feelings and your emotions. Your breath is closely connected to your emotions. Begin to make observations in this territory; we will delve into deeper realms in a later chapter.*

9. *Continue noticing your breath as you are standing, and gradually begin to walk. When you feel comfortable walking, increase your speed and try running, and other ways of moving, like*

skipping, dancing, jumping, jogging, or crawling. Notice if and how your breath changes. Are you still extending your exhale? Are your ribs moving three-dimensionally? Can you walk and run and not interfere with your breathing? Can you still exhale completely to get your reflex inhale?

10. *If you're in a group, meet someone, or if you're working by yourself, imagine meeting someone. Stop and talk to that person. Notice what happens to your breath during the interaction.*

11. *Take on another character as you move, and explore their movement. Notice the character's breath. What are his or her breathing tendencies and patterns?*

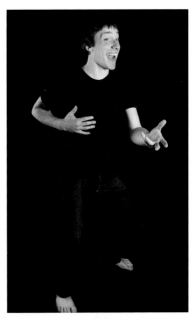

Exploring the breath and movement of a character.

12. *As you develop and explore different characters, you will find that different breathing patterns emerge. For example, if your character is depressed, they will probably collapse down in the chest. You will find that does not allow your ribs to move very much. As you continue to breathe this way, you can notice how the rest of you is affected. How do you feel? How do you see? How do you move? What drives you? What is your mood? Is your rhythm different? Your whole being is transformed when a breathing pattern is changed.*

Exploring the breath of a character is very powerful work. It can create such nuance in the role. On exploring the breath work of a character, one student said, "I was asked to think of a character's needs and let that inform my breath. I chose Dave from Devil's Teacup. I thought of how much Dave needs Max to leave and why. That is when I found Dave's breath. From the character's breathing pattern, the full embodiment of the character's body emerged, and everything I did was informed from there. The entire character came to life from starting with the breath."

Breath and Sensation on Stage

When you are on stage, sometimes you are standing or sitting very close to another actor. What happens to your breath?

Exercise to Explore Breath and Sensation on Stage

This is a set of exercises for two or more people. You can do this exercise with a partner or with a group. Try them first as yourself, then as your character.

Part 1:

1. *In a large space, walk around the stage or rehearsal room and weave in and out of one another.*
2. *If you get close to someone else, notice if you hold your breath. If you do, what happens to your whole body?*
3. *Make the moving space smaller.*
4. *When the circle is smaller and you are closer together, do you breathe? Does your breath get shorter? Quicker?*

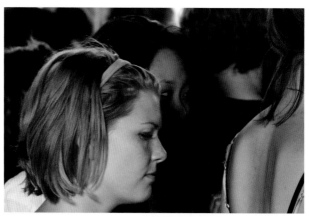

Exploring breath and sensation in a small circle.

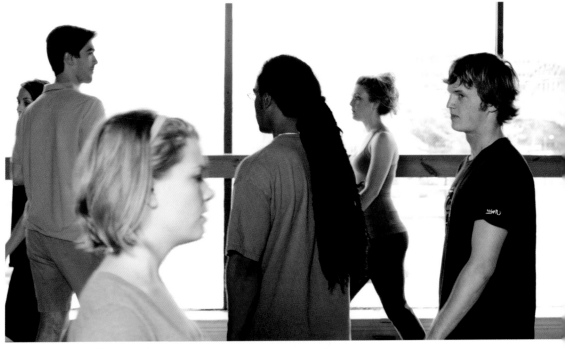

Exploring breath and sensation in a large circle.

5. *Make the circle bigger again. Is it easier to breathe now? When it is easier to breathe, what happens to your whole body? Are you more relaxed? At ease?*

6. *Explore the space being closer together again, and then farther apart. Notice what happens as you make changes in the size of the space, and move closer to, and farther away from, other people. Can you move and be close to someone else and breathe with ease?*

Part 2:

Preparation: *Take a moment here and notice how your breathing pattern can be influenced by other people, and specifically either positively or negatively influenced by people who you are comfortable with and not. When you stand next to someone you feel comfortable and resonate with, your breathing pattern is different than when you stand next to someone you do not feel comfortable with or resonate with. Let's now notice what these differences are by naming the sensations that occur inside your body as you approach and retreat from various people.*

1. *Do the exploration again (moving close to one another and farther apart) and name sensations that occur in your body when you stop breathing, or as you come close to someone else.*

Your body may experience sensations that may include feeling fluttery, contracted, queasy, frozen, spacey, dense, energized, expansive, tingly, electric, bubbly, buzzy, shaky, floating, sweaty, dizzy, fluid, and so on.

2. *Do the exploration again (moving close to one another and farther apart) and name sensations you feel in your body when you start breathing again as you are farther apart.*

Part 3:

1. *Give basic directions for suspension and support.*

- *Allow my feet to be on the ground.*
- *Allow the ground to support me.*
- *Allow my ankles, knees, and hips to be open to receive the support.*
- *Allow the support from the ground to come up through my legs, spine, and head.*
- ***Allow myself to breathe, and notice the room.***
- *Allow my neck to be free.*
- *Allow my head to free forward and up, or away from my spine.*
- *Allow my back to lengthen and widen.*
- *Allow my shoulders to widen, and my arms to free out of my back.*

- *Allow my ribs to move with my breath on my sternum and spine, as I notice the room.*

2. *Repeat Part 1 of the exercise, and then Part 2, starting from the place of having given your basic directions. Notice if there are any differences in your breathing patterns or any emotions that come up.*

When you are directing and you are aware of your feet on the ground and the ground supporting you, notice how your breathing and sensations change as you approach someone. When you are directed and more present with yourself, you can stay with your self and your breathing and not be thrown off so easily by the presence of another whether you feel comfortable with them or not. I believe that when you are directed, breathing, and in yourself, you have what I call **"the kind of support that no one can take away."**

After doing this exercise, one student commented, "When I feel the full capacity of my breath, I don't need to apologize for anything." In other words, when he does not have his full breath, he feels inadequate and needs to apologize. Our full breath can give us our full sense of an expanded self, with no apologies necessary.

Explore your own breathing patterns both on stage and off with these exercises. Know what happens to your optimal breath and reflex inhale as you walk onto the stage or the set, put on your makeup, or take a curtain call. Know for yourself what interferes with your normal breathing cycle.

I believe proper breathing can make a huge difference in the quality and length of an actor's career. Proper breath calms, energizes, and circulates oxygen, promoting health and emotional well-being. As you are able to choose to use your respiratory system with improved coordination and attention, you have more vitality on and off the set or stage.

CHAPTER 7

Trauma

Trauma is a word that means different things to different people. An event that may be overwhelming to one person may not bother somebody else. Dropping the ice cream off a newly acquired ice cream cone can be devastating to a young child, but to an adult it's probably just more of a nuisance. An event such as a divorce may cripple one person and may seemingly hardly affect another.

Trauma occurs when the bodily systems are faced with situations they cannot handle. The nervous system can be overwhelmed with an accident or a horrific event such as a rape or a murder. The digestive system cannot deal with food poisoning or swallowing large amounts of water in a near-drowning incident. The heart and circulatory system do not function well with heartbreak or loss of a loved one. The respiratory system cannot function well at certain altitudes or when the air quality is low because of smoke or pollutants. **For my explanations and exercises, the concept of trauma includes any situation that is overwhelming or difficult.** Trauma may be a deficit attunement (some kind of lack of communication) in the environment, or a disturbed rhythm between two people. It can even be someone slamming a door behind you that startles you. Traumas can be from things that happened when you were young, in the womb even, or an upsetting event that happened to you earlier in the day.

In our society we tend to put overwhelming and traumatic experiences away and forget about them. **But they don't actually go away: the body remembers them.** The body remembers and tells the story. Traumatic experiences stored in the body affect how you use yourself. An actor on stage or screen has two choices: use what is already happening habitually in the body, or become aware and make a change. For example, if you have a lot of anxiety for one reason or another, you can play characters that are anxious, enacting them well with fidgeting and nervous ticks that are your own anxious habits. Or you can look into your personal anxiety patterns and change them, and then be able to play characters with a variety of physical habits.

I was working with an actor who told me that she always clenched her right fist. She said she had now learned to unclench her fist as a voluntary act, but that it always clenched again. I asked her if she ever had an injury to her right hand, but she said not. I asked her if she ever had a fall or a car accident where she may have braced herself with her right hand; she said not. I told my student that hands do not just clench out of the blue for no reason. I asked her if she'd had any trauma in her life, and she said, "No, nothing unusual." Unable to find an answer, I decided to move on to something else. But a few moments later, the young woman remembered, "Oh, when I was four years old, I had an operation on my back. Oh, it was on my right side. And, oh: I almost died." There we had found our answer to her clenched right fist. Even though she did not consider back surgery and almost dying a traumatic experience, I did. That surgery was not in her conscious awareness, but her body remembered the experience. The habit of clenching her right hand interfered with her stage presence. This is just one of many examples of traumatic events that we may not consciously think of but that affect our body in everyday life as well as the process of playing a role on stage.

Oftentimes when I am working with an actor, an unusual image or pattern of tension will emerge. When we take the time to explore it and follow it through, we usually find that the pattern connects to some overwhelming life incident. Marla was having a hard time singing a few lines in her mostly speaking role. She felt darkness come over her as she began to sing. It did not take too much tracking and exploration before she realized that her second-grade teacher had told her, "You can't sing well."

Tracking

The process of paying attention to the sensations in your body is called tracking. Tracking engages the felt sense, or the ability to feel sensations, inside your body. If you live with your awareness mostly in your head, like most people do, and are not used to paying attention to your body, you may find tracking difficult at first. As you pay attention to your body, you might say that you don't feel anything. But as you continue to pay attention, you may start to notice small things, like slight temperature changes, contractions, trembling, other small movements, or eventually, weight changes. This process of tracking sensations can be helpful when overwhelming feelings arise.

As you learn to pay attention to these feelings, which are usually triggered stored feelings or traumas from the past, you can then listen to your body and let the feelings be heard. As you pay attention to the sensation, you can allow yourself also to be aware of the present moment, feeling your feet connecting to the ground or your sitting bones on the chair, which then may provide some sense of relief. **Going back and forth from the overwhelming sensation to connecting to a pleasant sensation in the present moment is a process called pendulating.** Eventually, after pendulating back and forth between the stored traumatic sensation of the past and the present feeling of being connected to yourself and the moment, the sensation will start to subside, and might eventually even go away. Levine explains that "pendulation is the primal rhythm expressed as movement from constriction to expansion—and back to constriction, but gradually opening to more and more expansion."[1]

I was working with a nineteen-year-old on getting in and out of a chair. The young woman weighed no more than eighty pounds.

Yet as we worked, she kept saying how heavy she felt, and began to cry. As I helped her explore those feelings and taught her better use, she soon got very light under my hands, and stopped crying. We pendulated back and forth a few times between the heavy and the light feelings, and the heavy feeling eventually subsided. After the lesson, she told me that she had a long history of eating disorders. In the work we did, she realized that she always felt heavy, so she did not want to eat. When she gave her directions, and began to change her use, she began to feel light. She became aware of suspension and support, and felt the kinesthetic lightness, the floating quality. It was a very eye-opening experience for her that she did not need to feel so heavy.

Tracking Your Sensations Exercises

Preparation: *Sit in a comfortable chair. Find a place where you feel safe.*

1. *Feel your body as a container. It contains your thoughts, emotions, organs, and more.*
2. *Notice this container, and your skin or clothing, touching the chair. It may feel soft or scratchy or sticky.*
3. *Notice that the chair supports you. Your spine touches the back, and your sitting bones touch the seat. The body needs support and containment.*
4. *Sense your internal organs, especially your belly. What is going on in your belly? Is it flaccid or constricted? Any butterflies? Is your heart soft or tight?*
5. *Every time you have a thought, your body has a sensation. Explore different thoughts: "I am enjoying this sunny day." What happens in your body? "I know this person betrayed me." What happens in your body? "Everything in my life is going perfectly." "My husband lost his job." "I'm hungry." "I'm in love." Track what happens in your body.*

6. *It is important to be able to find a sensation in your body that feels good or comfortable, like warmth or expansion. If that is not possible, find a spot that feels less troubled.*

7. *As you do the tracking, you may notice that the sensation (for example, shaking) appears for a few moments, then disappears, and there is a breath of relief. Then the sensation appears again. The pendulating back and forth between the sensation and the sense of calm may continue until eventually the symptom subsides. You can pendulate between any discomfort—like shaking—and any sensation of comfort—like expansion. This helps your body restore its natural rhythm.*

8. *You can also practice tracking your sensations by guiding your thinking to different parts of your body and becoming aware of the sensations that exist there. You can begin with the joints in your extremities and work your way to your torso. Begin sensing your feet, including your toes and ankles; then move up to sense your knees and hips, and your lower torso. Notice if there are any changes as a result of this sensing—perhaps less constriction and more flow in your legs and lower body. Let your whole body know these changes have occurred. Now follow the same process with your arms: hands, fingers, wrists, elbows, and shoulders, into your chest, neck, and head. Does your breath change? Are there any changes in your arms and upper body? Integrate these changes into your whole body.*

Some bodily sensations that you might experience in any of these exercises may include feeling flowing, tingly, numb, fluid, spacious, knotted, energized, breathless, trembling, sweaty, or icy.

As you practice the Tracking Your Sensations Exercise, you will become more adept at identifying your own sensations and those of your character. Your sensations affect your use. When you feel knotted in your shoulder, your use in your upper body will most likely be contracted and compressed. On the other hand, when you feel energized and flowing, your use tends to be buoyant and upright.

James was in a show that had only two actors. He was on stage the whole time, with many lines to speak. Before each show, the thought of the whole performance felt daunting, and he found himself getting very anxious. He felt his heart pounding before the curtain went up. He told me, "I began to do the Tracking Your Sensations Exercise, just being with the pounding in my heart. I began to settle a little. Then, as I started to pendulate between the pounding and the relief, I realized that I could use the other actor on stage as relief to ground me. Every time I felt a wave of anxiety, I grounded myself in the other actor. It was amazing."

Boundaries

Once you are able to track your sensations, you can be more aware of your personal boundaries. There is a degree of comfort or discomfort that is felt when someone stands or moves close to you. Of course, this may vary depending on your trauma history. Often in trauma, a boundary has been broken. Someone or something that you did not want or expect came into your personal space. It is clear in the animal kingdom that a creature knows when danger approaches. Humans also have this ability to detect when danger is near. When you are comfortable and resonate with someone, a friend, it is different than standing close to a stranger at the bus stop. This exercise helps you identify your habitual pattern of comfort with proximity.

Exercise to Explore Boundaries

This exercise can be done with a real or imagined partner.

Preparation: *Stand in a room in a comfortable and safe space. Place a string or piece of twine on the floor around you in a circle to define "your space," with a diameter of four to six feet.*

1. *Start by asking your partner to stand a comfortable distance away from you, maybe six to ten feet. You may notice that this is farther away than you imagined. Notice what happens in your body.*

2. *Tell your partner to take one step closer. Check to see if it feels comfortable.*

3. *Continue to tell your partner to step closer until it is uncomfortable. What happens when he or she approaches the string of "your" space? You may feel a slight contraction somewhere in your body or a wave of anxiety. When you do, tell him or her to stop moving forward.*

4. *Have your partner approach from the front, the back, and both sides. Notice which direction is most comfortable, and which is least comfortable.*

Just begin to notice where your personal boundaries are. We will learn in later exercises what to do about them.

Obviously, when you are on stage or set with someone, no matter what you feel, you need to be able to go on with your scene. But this exercise can be helpful for you to understand your own reaction and responses to physical proximity. This exercise helps awaken your kinesthetic sense. Are you more aware of the space around you and your boundaries? You can begin to wonder what kind of boundary a certain character may have.

"Be With"

Life has challenges and discomforts in all shapes and sizes. These can range from a nagging pain in your shoulder to a major illness like cancer or heart disease. We all know that the body has a built-in immune system to fight disease. When you get a cut, you do not need to "do" anything; the body will heal the cut. This same healing principle is available with other discomforts when they are brought to awareness.

Often, when you have an uncomfortable situation, you want to get rid of the discomfort. If you feel pain in your shoulder, you want it to go away. But viewed in a different light, we can learn that the discomfort in your shoulder is telling you that something is off in your system, and that something wants attention.

The body is a highly attuned instrument, and it is very sensitive. Rather than ignoring these signs, learn to pay attention to them, and you will be able to improve them accordingly. If you pay attention to the discomforts and become curious about them, they can shift. **This process is called self-regulation.** With no awareness, there is less possibility for change. But once you bring your awareness to a situation, it is as if your body says, "Are you sure you want to be holding that muscle?" With your new awareness, you can say no, and the pain can actually shift. The body will often regulate itself back to homeostasis, or equilibrium, when you are able to "be with" the discomfort. We saw an example of this in chapter 1 with Carol, who was able to "be with" the tightness in her chest, which allowed the tightness to shift without her having to do anything else.

Exercise to "Be With"

Preparation: *Find a comfortable, quiet place to sit or lie down, where you won't be disturbed.*

1. *Be with an overwhelming emotion. For example, you might say, "I have a show tonight that I'm anxious about." Sometimes*

emotions take over, and it feels like you are only that emotion and nothing else.

2. *Pay close attention to your body. Where do you feel the emotion in your body? In your chest, belly, back, arms?*

3. *Once you have located the emotion, take a moment to look at it and see what it feels like. If you are anxious, you may feel a fluttering in your chest or a churning in your stomach.*

4. *Now separate the emotion from the physical sensation. See the physical sensation as separate from the emotion. As I stated in step 1, the emotion of anxiety tends to take over your whole body-mind awareness. You must now work to separate them. You are not only your anxiety.*

5. *Explore the physical sensation and describe it. For example, I feel a fluttering, like butterfly wings moving in the breeze. Describe the sensations very specifically. The more you can describe it, almost like you are a witness, the more you are separate from it, allowing it to change.*

6. *Notice if there are any changes. Does the flapping get bigger? Stronger? Does it feel like the flaps are now creating waves in the ocean? Or does the flapping slow down and feel more calming, inspiring a deep breath?*

7. *Integrate these changes into your whole body. Let your whole body understand that a change has taken place, and let it assimilate the change. For example, now you might feel less fluttering, less tension, and less overall anxiety. Allow the process of self-regulation to return you to a state of equilibrium.*

As you explore or repeat the Exercise to "Be With," you may want to inquire into:

- *Is this familiar?*
- *How old do I feel?*
- *Does it remind me of any specific instances from the past?*
- *If I was fine a minute ago, what changed all of a sudden? Was*

it something from outside? Did someone say something? Or was it something my mind brought up for some reason?

- *What put me over the edge?*
- *Am I doing something that I wasn't aware of that is allowing this discomfort?*

One student complained that her shoulders were always tight and hurting, especially on stage. As she sat, I noticed that her feet were not resting flat on the floor, but lifted onto the lower bar of her chair. She told me that she could never keep her feet on the ground. She said that no matter how hard she tried, her feet always wanted to pull up. I asked her to just "be with" the feeling of always holding her feet up. I asked if she had any traumatic experiences. She said no. After a few moments her face lit up. "When I was eight years old, I fell off the monkey bars, but it was no big deal." I asked, "Did you fall backward?" She said, "Yes." I said, "Maybe it was a bigger deal than you thought." I asked her to stay with the feelings of that fall, and her legs coming up as she fell back off the monkey bars. As she was being with these sensations, her nervous system shifted, and her feet dropped to the ground. She said, "My toes aren't numb anymore. I feel a breath of fresh air, like I'm coming outside for the first time." From that moment forward, she began to sit with her feet on the ground, and her shoulders were finally able to drop, in her personal life and on stage. She felt awake and alive.

The Exercise to "Be With" can be used without knowing what the traumatic event might have been. "As I was playing a Shakespearean king in difficult circumstances," said another student, "I had a lot of neck and jaw tension. I kept trying to stretch it out. I was judging the feeling of tension. 'I am going to fix this,' I said to myself. Then I decided to try the 'be with' exercise. I had no conceived notion of what this tension was. I was just going to be with it. My neck and jaw released by themselves. I didn't do anything. My jaw says thank-you to this exercise."

In both of these examples, the student was able to connect to the discomfort or fear, and not try to get rid of it. Trying to ignore or get rid of pain, or to hold down and not feel feelings, takes a lot of work both muscularly and energetically. When you stop this work, there is an increase in energy. The body is then available to respond more appropriately and more fully to the moment. Little by little you get comfortable with having more energy in your body to speak, move, or express yourself.

The Exercise to "Be With" may seem hard to believe. First of all, who wants to be with pain? You just want to get rid of it! And second, who believes that being with discomfort is going to shift it? But after you see that attempts to get rid of pain don't actually work, you may want to explore another approach. Be with what is. You have to accept a problem in order to change it. Rejecting what is really going on and not acknowledging it only keeps you blocked, unable to make changes for improvement.

Stuck

When you are unable to progress for one reason or another, you are stuck. You can be stuck in yourself or stuck in the role you are playing. "Stuck" may be a habitual pattern for you that prevents your innate talent from blossoming. Or you may feel stuck, but it's actually a faulty sensory perception, and you may not be as stuck as you feel. A stuck feeling can manifest in many forms, including mental, physical, emotional, or spiritual. Being mentally stuck can feel like, "I just cannot think of a way to solve this problem." Physically stuck can look like, "I just cannot walk the way my character walks." Emotionally stuck may be always feeling anger. Spiritually stuck may be feeling lost and disconnected from the world around you. Feeling stuck in any of these areas can feel like there's a barrier blocking your progress in life, and it's a dilemma that needs attention.

What can you do when you feel stuck emotions with yourself or with your character? Or what do you do when there is a role that you are cast in that you cannot seem to get? What if you are working on a play and you feel stuck in the development of your character's journey? All of these situations can feel overwhelming and uncomfortable, like something does not fit right.

Stuck or difficult states show up. **They are often parts of yourself trying to communicate or to show you something.** To find the root cause of the barrier, you need to take time and slow things down. You need to create a distance so that you can step outside your experience and simply observe yourself and say: "I am here as a witness, watching this stuck feeling." You also need to turn down the volume of the experience that is overwhelming you. You can't see what's there if you have too many thoughts and feelings swirling around. As a witness, you slow things down by stepping outside the situation for a moment, so that you can see each tiny thought, feeling, and body sensation as it is happening.

This practice is not a way to get rid of anything, change anything, or have your experience be different. It's merely a way to allow yourself to be with what is going on and to initiate a relationship toward it. You want to have an interest in it, and be curious about it. Then when you know what the stuck feeling is really about, what's happening on a deeper level, you can deal with the issue accordingly.

Exercise to Explore a Stuck Place

Preparation: *Prepare yourself for lying-down work.*

1. *The first step of exploring a stuck place is to be with whatever is going on. "I am overwhelmed and feel like I cannot move." "I feel no energy." Whatever comes up, just be with it. Do not try to get rid of it. As you are exploring your stuck place, you may want to inquire into:*

- *Is this familiar?*
- *How old do I feel?*
- *Does it remind me of any specific instances from the past?*
- *If I was fine a minute ago, what changed all of a sudden? Was it something from outside? Did someone say something? Or was it something my mind brought up for some reason?*
- *What put me over the edge?*

Your stuck place may actually change just by being with it. As we have seen, the body-mind system is wired for well-being and self-regulation. When you have unconscious negative thoughts or feelings, they can wreak havoc on your mind and body. But when you become aware of them, sometimes they can automatically shift. If you feel an inward shift and the feelings go away, that's great. And if you find things don't shift, don't judge yourself; it's okay. You can learn a lot from exploring the stuck place.

2. *Witness the stuck place and recognize that it is not the whole of you. It is only a part. As you know, when these parts take over, it can feel in the moment like that is all that exists, but as you step back to witness them, you can see the separateness. For example, a stuck place may be "I didn't get the role." In the moment it feels like "I'm not good enough." But the whole of you knows "I'm a good actor and I will get another role."*

3. *Take a moment and notice where this stuckness lives inside you. Is it in your chest? Or is it in your arms or legs? Trauma often gets stuck in the joints, especially the knees.* **What is the experience behind the symptom?** *Perhaps if you notice it in your heart, your heart will feel heavy, or if in your knees, your knees will feel weak.*

4. *What color is it? Does it have a shape? Are there words that go with it? Is there any movement that it makes?*

5. *Take that internal experience and imagine it in front of you, outside your body.*

6. *Now take a look at it. What happens inside you as you see it outside of yourself? Are you able to be curious and interested? If you hate it, it may not want to open to you, or reveal itself to you. Take some time and interact with this image. Ask it what it wants you to know. You might need to spend some time with this step, being as understanding and open as possible.*

7. *There will likely be a small change in your body or breathing, like a sense of relief, a breath, a yawn, a wave of energy. Allow your whole body to integrate the new feeling. Let your arms and legs know that a change has taken place.*

8. *After you have worked on your own stuck place, choose a character you are working on and see his or her stuck place. Is it the same as yours? Where does the character meet the self?*

Often the pattern will pendulate back and forth a few times between the holding and the release. For example, a student once felt her stuck place as a brick wall surrounding her body. As she paid attention to the image, it started to shift. A breath followed. Then the image of the brick wall changed and morphed into a wooden wall. As she stayed with that, another breath followed. Then it appeared as a paper wall, and eventually it disappeared.

One student, Joe, was having trouble in his show; he was working hard to make his character believable. He felt stuck. When we started working together privately, he said his breathing felt restricted, his bottom ribs could not release, and his breath would not go below his lower ribs. He felt like he could not get a full breath. His realized that his ribs were stuck, and he had been trying to figure out what was causing the restriction. I told him to pay attention to his lower ribs, and try to discover what was actually happening. He took a moment to observe his lower ribs. After a few minutes of paying attention to what was going on in his body, his ribs began to drop lower, and his neck released.

He then said, "I feel unrestricted and unstuck." He realized that he had been trying to figure out the restriction and manipulate it into something else, instead of being with it. As he was being with his stuck place, he felt his underarm release as his breath opened. Before he had been concentrating on trying to breathe, but in the process of trying so hard, was not allowing himself to breathe. The key was staying with the stuck place, which was the restriction at the bottom of Joe's ribs. As the restriction began to disintegrate, and he was breathing more fully, I asked him "What do you notice about the room?" "It's there," he exclaimed. "And the room is part of my being. . . . I feel alive and able to sense things around me. . . . No question of stoppage." Joe was able to translate this experience into his show. Playing the role of a businessman, he was now able to feel relaxed and easy in the role.

After learning the principles of the trauma work, another acting student said, "As I did my scene, I was able to find my power and the free flow of emotions despite the physical limitations of being tied up in a chair. I was also able to absorb physical violence and emotional trauma during the scene and use the work I learned from Betsy to bring myself out of those circumstances after the scene was over, which is imperative with a scene like that. The use of this technique both to bring myself to the work and, in particular, to separate the work from my life, is a priceless tool that I can already tell will enable me to do this work for a lifetime."

As you can see, the trauma work opens new avenues for deep change. It gives you access to aspects of yourself that are below your conscious awareness. I imagine that you never thought that a minor fall in the past could be restricting your body today. I find that if an actor is willing and able to track his or her inner sensations, and process them as I have explained above, then there are great benefits to be reaped: a less tense body, a freer voice, clearer thinking, and more.

As we end the "Principles" section, I hope you have begun to incorporate these ideas and practices into your artistic and daily life. Has your use changed? Are you able to breathe more fully more often? Are you more aware of your inner sensations? These exercises can release infinite creative potential on your journey to an expanded self.

Part Two
PREPARATION

CHAPTER 8

Presence and Inhibition

When you think about it, the present moment is the only actual real, all-inclusive moment that we have. All senses can potentially respond accurately to the moment. The other states of awareness are imaginings of what might be or what has been. However, because of past overwhelming experiences that are biologically incomplete and still stuck in the body (as we read about in chapter 7 on trauma), what seems to be the present is actually clouded over, or veiled, by experiences of the past. We must learn to be able to tell the difference between the actual present moment and our projection of the past onto it, and then to live and respond in the present moment.

Presence

To be in the present moment is to be aware of yourself and your environment in this moment. Somehow, we often forget to be present. We tend to think about the past and the future: "what he said" or "what you are going to say." In reality, the past is gone, and the future has not happened yet. The more you are in the present, the more you understand its value.

The best investment for your time and energy is the present. Your senses are alive with information in each moment. Become aware of your body and your surroundings. You fully inhabit your body, and you can make choices about how you are using yourself. Allow yourself to participate in the present and just be. The present is ongoing. Try to stay with it and experience each moment. The ongoing present consists of this moment . . . then this moment . . . then this moment, and so on.

Most people move through life with attention focused either outside themselves through perception, or inside themselves through what is called proprioception. **Proprioception** comes from the Latin *proprio*, meaning "one's own." It is the sense that includes information about what is happening inside your body, such as indicating whether the body is moving with the required effort, and also informing you what is happening at your joints, and where the various parts of the body are located in relation to one another.

For example, you are working on your computer with all your attention outside of yourself and on the computer screen. A few hours later, you realize your back hurts. All of your attention then goes inside you to feel your back, and you forget what you were working on at the computer. When all of your attention focuses either outside you or inside you, you do not experience a connection between the inner and the outer worlds. To be present, you want to explore the balance of your inner and outer awareness. Try to be present with fifty percent of your attention outward and fifty percent of your attention inward, which I call your **"50-50 awareness."** This way of being present allows you to make correlations between the inner and outer worlds as they happen. This is very important for an actor to understand in order to be able to create believable characters on stage. Actors have to stay connected to who they are, who their character is, and also be aware of the sets and the other actors on stage.

Another element that might interfere with the balance of perception and proprioception is something called **"endgaining."** When you are doing a task like working at your computer, you often are going one hundred percent for the end product of the work. This would be one hundred percent perception—totally involved in your computer—and would include very little presence in your surroundings. In this case, you are doing your computer work and not paying attention to how you do it, or how your body is included. Rather than just being focused on the outcome of the work and endgaining, try to remember the 50-50 awareness, and include attention to your body as you work.

The role that presence plays on stage is paramount. It seems like such a simple task just to be present on stage. Being present is a simple task, but it is not always an easy one. Outside factors such as fear and worry ("Who's in the audience tonight?") or thinking about the future ("What am I going to eat after the show?") can take you out of being in the present moment. But when you can allow yourself to be present on stage, your body is alive and vibrant. You have awareness of what is happening inside your body. You are acutely aware of what is happening around you, in the larger environment, and with fellow actors. You are aware of your suspension and support. Presence is a practice that gives you infinite creative potential—not just in rehearsal, but also in daily life.

The present moment is a still point in a turning world. The present moment has a quality of stillness to it that is very important for an actor to understand. From presence and stillness you can give and receive. From this stillness you can listen to your fellow actors, and get what you need from your scene partner to help you move through the scene. My colleague, the acting professor Judy Braha, says, "The answer is in the other person." When you are present and listening, you get that answer.

The talented Hollywood actor Heath Ledger once said, "The Alexander Technique helps me to burrow into roles like gay cowboys and drug addicts by focusing on my posture, movement, and presence."[1] This suggests the effectiveness of the practice of presence in order to deeply connect to the inner and outer life of a character.

Exercise for Balancing Inner and Outer Attention, Your 50-50 Awareness

Being present is a part of many practices, such as Pilates, yoga, and meditation. My unique approach to presence has to do with exploring the balance of inner and outer attention—of learning to focus half of your attention inward to your body, and half outward to the environment. This way, wherever your attention goes inside your body, you take the environment with you, and when your attention goes out to your surroundings, your inner experience goes with you.

Preparation: *Let's start with the ever-popular activity of sitting at your computer.*

1. *Sit at your computer and start typing in your habitual way. Do you have any awareness of your use, or what your body is doing? Are you breathing? Is your neck pulled back? Or tilted downward? Are your wrists held tight? Allow the information from your body to come to you.*

2. *Now type something, paying fifty percent of your attention to inside your body and fifty percent of your attention to your computer and your environment. What do you notice now? Perhaps more of a sense of your whole body in relationship to the room, including the computer?*

3. *As you sit at your computer, take into account how you are using yourself. Is your back held stiffly? Are your shoulders tense? Might you be creating back pain for yourself?*

4. *While still keeping part of your awareness within, and part without, try giving your basic directions as you bring your attention to the top of your spine, and to your sitting bones on the chair:*
   - *Allow my neck to be free.*
   - *Allow my head to free forward and up, or away from my spine.*

- *Allow my back to lengthen and widen.*
- *Allow my shoulders to widen.*
- *Allow my ribs to move with my breath on my sternum and spine.*
- *Allow my knees to release forward and away.*
- *Allow my feet to be on the ground.*
- *Allow the ground and the chair to support me.*
- *Allow the support from the ground to come up through my legs, spine, and head.*
- *Allow myself to breathe.*

5. *Do you feel different after giving your directions? What is your relationship to your computer now? Try typing a few words. Are you able to focus on what you are typing, and to pay attention to your use and what is going on with your body?*

Many people tend to live only in their thinking minds. The 50-50 Awareness exercise helps you expand your idea of presence to include what is happening in your body and the world around you. As you learn to become aware of yourself and your surroundings, presence becomes an all-inclusive moment that allows your mind to observe details and not think about them or try to figure them out. You can just be present and have an expanded field of attention.

Exercise to Explore Presence

Preparation: *To prepare to explore presence, stand in the middle of the room you're in. Take a moment to establish your 50-50 awareness. This exercise will help you begin to develop the courage and stamina to be present with whatever is going on.*

1. *Look around the room. Let your eyes be free to wander.*
2. *Notice three things about the room. Describe them in detail out loud or to yourself. This brings you to the present moment. When you take in the environment and see specifics in the*

moment, there is less chatter in your mind, and you can be present. You are capturing the chattering mind by describing the details, and overriding it from needing to wander. For example: As I look at the wall, I can say, "I see the wood grain in the trim. It has squiggly lines running through it. I see the shiny brass handle on the door," and so on. "As I do the exercise, my mind is focused in the present moment, and I am connected both inwardly to myself, and to the outer world." This experience of presence can create a sense of wonder for seemingly mundane moments.

The chattering mind usually jumps around from thought to thought, obsessing about the past and worrying about the future. To capture and train the mind, you need to focus on your present activity. In a world of multitasking, this can be a challenging endeavor. But stick with it. Focusing on the present can be an invaluable tool in your acting work and in your life because connecting with the present refreshes each moment for you to feel more awake and alive.

> *3. In addition to "describing the details," you can also try watching your breath. This technique is often used in yoga and meditation, and it's very helpful for honing the mind and quieting thoughts. To watch your breath, focus on the air coming in and then feel the air go out. Do this for a few rounds. As you watch your breath, continue to balance your inner and outer awareness. As you breathe, you are present with your breath and your body, aware of yourself, aware of the world around you, fully present in the given moment.*

One student wrote about her experience of presence in class. "For the past few weeks I have been feeling very unfocused and generally confused about the apathetic nature of my thoughts. When I would tell myself to 'be present,' my mind seemed to race even more out of control, to the point that giving up and ignoring my state seemed to be the only option. However, I was miserable in this way, and continued to hope that I would wake up the next day with a clear mind.

"When I brought up this issue in class, I realized that I was really meant to work from where I am. Betsy asked me to stay with the confusion of my mind and recognize what it felt like. As I stayed present, sat with the confusion, and allowed my frustrating apathy to simmer, suddenly my left heel jumped off of the floor. My Achilles tendon had been bothering me for about a week, and I had been choosing to ignore the pain. When I was present in class in front of everyone and my foot jumped up, I couldn't ignore it anymore. It was like a clue, a red flag sent from my body into my mental consciousness saying, 'Hey! Hello! I'm here right now in this moment, please pay attention to me.' As I paid attention to my foot, my mind settled and became clearer.

"I learned that the body and the mind are truly two parts of the same system that knows how to balance itself out. Ultimately, the greatest lesson is to work from where I am. Being present isn't necessarily about being totally 'Zenned out' with only a complete awareness of the world around me, but being present must also include what is going on with me, 50-50 awareness."

Exercise to Explore Presence on Stage

This exercise can be done in any rehearsal space or practice room to prepare for stage work. **When you do this exercise, try to discover the difference between concentrating and narrowing to convey an idea versus paying attention to yourself and your environment to convey an idea.** We are taught that concentrating is a good thing to do, but for most people this includes a narrowing of attention. That narrowing causes you to not be present with everything else that might be going on. The exercise here is about allowing your attention to include your surroundings, rather than excluding them.

1. *Stand or sit in your chosen space, allowing the ground to support you as you prepare to speak a line or make a movement. Do a few silent "la la las" (from the Exercise to Explore Extending the Exhale).*
2. *Become aware of the space around you: the stage, the set, and so on. Don't focus or concentrate on the activity of speaking or moving and thus narrow in. Instead, notice the room: above you, below you, in front of you, in back of you, and to your sides. Remember your 50-50 awareness.*
3. *Allow your body-mind to open to this expanded field of attention. Now try speaking the line or making a movement. How does that feel different than your initial impulse to do the action?*
4. *Fully experience your awareness of yourself in relationship to the room or stage. Because your consciousness fills the room, you are larger, and you do not have to "try," by pushing or tightening, to fill the space. This kind of presence includes your awareness of inner and outer balance. Can you feel your expanded field of attention?*

One actor I worked with had to run onto the stage for her scene. She was feeling uncomfortable with her arrival as she was focusing and narrowing her attention to try to fit into the ongoing scene. She did the presence work, taking in the entire space and sensing the space above, below, and all around her before she ran in. She said, "I ran like I was flying and had wings, and I was launched into the given imaginary circumstances of the play without trying."

This exercise can also be very helpful for stage fright. I was once working with an actor in a master class who became very nervous attempting to perform a monologue. She was concentrating intensely on saying the words correctly, but had limited awareness of herself and the whole room. She felt small, and the audience seemed large and daunting. Once I walked her through this exercise, she became aware of the whole room, including the four corners, and especially the back wall. This made her feel bigger, and she filled the space with her presence. The audience of the other actors happened to be in the space also, but they did not intimidate her. She was present in the given moment in space and time, causing her fears to dissipate and her nerves to subside. We will explore more about performance anxiety in later chapters.

Exercise to Explore Presence and Endgaining

1. *In a room with some space, choose to walk from point A to point B.*
2. *As you walk, notice how you do it. Are you leaning forward instead of remaining upright? Are you tensing your shoulders? Have you stopped breathing, or are you using too much tension? Is your mind wandering?*
3. *Now stop, and try walking the same path again, just being entirely present in the moment. You're just moving from A to B, not endgaining, pushing to get somewhere. Is your body less tense now? Are you not leaning forward? Is your mind present and in the moment, taking in the room?*
4. *Now try this exercise with other activities, such as picking up a book, preparing to sing a song, or even eating a cookie.*

When present with yourself, you can be aware of how you are doing what you are doing. The "how" is important. As stated earlier, **trying to get a specific job done, no matter what the consequences, is called endgaining.** With walking, endgaining may cause you to tighten more than necessary. With eating a cookie, endgaining may cause you to eat it too fast, hardly chewing and not even enjoying the taste. Endgaining can generate excessive muscular tension by your determination to get what you want, which causes you to not pay attention to yourself and the process of what you are doing. This can block you from getting optimal results. If you're rushing to get a job done and not paying attention to the process, you can end up making mistakes, or cause harm to yourself in the process.

Frank Pierce Jones quotes F. M. Alexander as saying, "No matter how many specific ends you may gain, you are worse off than before, [Alexander] maintained, if in the process of gaining them you have destroyed the integrity of the organism."[2] This is a powerful statement: by trying to do too much, the results can sometimes actually be detrimental.

The endgaining mode of behavior takes its toll. If you struggle to get something done and don't pay attention to the way you do it, you must then live with the results of the unconscious behavior. When you're not paying attention, you are not present. For example, if a director is giving you notes in rehearsal, and you are already thinking about the end of rehearsal and meeting up with your friends, you might miss pertinent information the director is trying to tell you. If you're not in the moment paying attention, it's very easy to miss not only what's going on around you but also bypass good use. When you're endgaining, you're not experiencing the present moment.

Exercise to Explore Endgaining on Stage

Preparation: *Find a monologue or a short piece of text that you'd like to explore.*

1. *Let yourself be present on a stage or in a performance space. Let your senses feel alive so that you see the seats in the house and hear the background sounds of the room.*
2. *Deliver your lines without endgaining. Use only as much effort as you need to convey the story. Make sure that you are not throwing your head back as you speak. Make sure you are keeping the experience of your whole body, your hips, your lower back, your legs, and your feet connected to the ground.*
3. *As you speak, can you feel the lack of excess tension? Can you*

feel the length of your back and the aim up along your spine?
Are you noticing new ideas and new perceptions emerging?

As we have seen, excessive muscular tension is usually generated with endgaining. In your determination to get what you want, you often block the results. On stage, when you "try" to get a laugh, you can block the natural impulses that arise that would be funny.

When you are present on stage, you allow your senses to speak to you. Your senses give you information about what comes to you. Let emotions come to you. Let the text come to you. You receive information from outside via your perception. This includes information about the other actor's words and actions as well as your environment. You receive information from inside yourself about feelings, tension, and impulses via your proprioception. This way you have a 50-50 awareness and can act on stage or on camera without endgaining in your performance.

One student experienced presence in her acting this way: "I was having trouble in *Under Milkwood* because everyone is on stage all the time. I found myself often starting to drift. The show really suffers if the ensemble on the sides is not engaged in actively listening. As I used my directions, I was able to stay present, and I was able to react genuinely to each moment."

Another student was having trouble being present and asked for my help. She said her mind and body felt disconnected, and that made her feel angry and frustrated, so she could not be present. I asked her what was happening in this present moment. She said, "I feel contracted. I'm not breathing, and I'm a seriously closed person." I asked her to notice what happened when she felt the contractions and the frustration. She said that her mind and body were beginning to work together and that she started to feel the tension release. She felt cooler and less angry. Then she said, "I feel present now. I can be me, instead of trying to be somebody else. When I try to be somebody else, I cannot be present."

Any kind of trying to be anything other than what is, takes you out of being in the present moment. Being present enhances your senses: it makes the colors of the world brighter, the smells and sounds clearer, and the textures more defined. Being fully present allows you to be your fully expanded self, which enlivens the space around you and can enhance your performance as you tell your story on stage or screen.

Inhibition—Nondoing

The practice of inhibition brings you into the present moment by suspending your habitual response. The habitual response is often anchored in the past and, as we have seen, often includes excess muscular tension. Remembering the exercise "Can I do less?" will help you permit the exiled parts to emerge as the habitual parts recede into the background. You then have a new choice as to how you use yourself.

Stage and screen actor Kevin Spacey was asked, "What is the best advice you have received from a director?" His response was: "Do it differently."[3] To do it differently, you must open the door to choice. This is what inhibition helps you achieve.

Inhibition, or nondoing, is the Actor's Secret. To respond with nonhabitual behavior, doing less can allow a totally different interpretation to surface. You tend to do what you think is right because you do not want to be wrong. But what if your idea of right is not right? If you keep doing what you think is right, you will not get to experience other choices. These other choices are unknown. Alexander used to say before teaching a lesson, "I must be willing to go into the unknown." The Alexander Technique presents a unique approach to responding to common stimuli. Alexander explained, "The act of refusing to respond, to the primary desire to gain an end, becomes the act of responding, volitionary act, to the conscious reasoned desire to employ the means whereby that end may be gained."[4] In other words, the act of refusing to respond becomes the act of responding. We can refuse to respond in a habitual way. This means saying no to the habit and saying yes to something else that may be unplanned or unknown. This is where you can find choice, being fully in the moment. Inhibiting the planned or habitual response helps you allow yourself to be fully present.

In acting, inhibition means not doing the immediate response. Let's say you are playing a character that you think is angry. Most likely, you approach the role with your idea of what angry looks and feels like—but that is what you do when you're angry. Instead, using inhibition, you can help yourself find the character's way of being angry. When you explore what it means for the character to be angry, try to feel your immediate habitual interpretation or response. Then, rather than immediately making that the choice for the way to play the character feeling angry, inhibit it, or stop. Then you can allow a new version of angry to emerge, something unique to the character. Maybe some other aspects of the character's given circumstances will come into play, making the character's version of angry different from your version of angry. No two people respond in exactly the same way, so by inhibiting, you allow your character to have his or her own unique version of angry rather than your habits of angry.

In some cases, you may discover that another emotion is actually in play besides anger. Something else might be going on that you had not seen because you were busy playing angry a certain way. Perhaps the character is actually scared, or sad, or both. You can even try inhibiting your character's habitual response. "Once I was working with a scene from Chekov's *Three Sisters,*" said a student, "where the character was playing anger. However, when I inhibited my habitual way of playing anger, there was hardly any anger. There was actually a lot of sadness in the scene." When the student inhibited his habitual response, a whole new element of the scene arose. Inhibiting your habitual responses makes way for new ideas, thoughts, and emotions to arise. This gives you a choice. It gives you freedom as an actor, and it gives you many more tools to work with.

I was sitting in on rehearsals for a play and noticed that one actor was playing a role the same way over and over. Later, we spoke, and I said to him, "Try doing the role in a way you have never done before." After he explored this aspect of inhibition, he said, "**I felt the freedom to not know what will happen.** It was very powerful." In the scene I had been watching, he had planned ideas about how he was going to explain his plans for his future to his mother. When he stopped talking to her in his preconceived way of how he thought the scene should go, something truthful and exciting emerged.

Often the question of spontaneity comes up when I introduce the concept of inhibition. **Many actors think that they are being spontaneous when what they are in fact doing is behaving habitually.** They are afraid of the moment of pause before the jump to their habitual response, that moment of inhibition and choice. They think that they are losing some kind of impulse, freedom, or momentum if they let themselves be fully present. In actuality, that pause before jumping to a habitual response, with proper attention, gives rise to many new possibilities that are formed in the moment, and choosing one of those is true spontaneity. This pause is the actor's great tool. This pause, which leads to choice, and to nonhabitual behavior, is the Actor's Secret.

After one of my classes on inhibition, a student said, "When I explored saying no to a habitual impulse, I found it very uncomfortable. But I made a decision to try it during a rehearsal for a show I was working on, *Macbeth*. I started listening in a new way, and really heard what Lady Macbeth was saying, and responded as if it was the first time I had heard it. In the scene, where I played Donalbain and find out that my father has been murdered, I used to plan an emotional response. This time I inhibited my usual response and listened and waited for more information. When he was described as bloody, I felt sick to my stomach, and tears began to swell, without me forcing them. I was truly in the moment."

This is an example of being present in the moment, stopping the habitual response, and choosing to be fully aware of the unfolding circumstances. This gave the student a visceral emotional response, which was spontaneous and appropriate to the situation.

Exercise to Explore Inhibition: The Three Choices

The Three Choices exercise is based on the format that Alexander used to change his habitual approach to speaking. Read through the complete explanation before exploring this exercise.

1. *Choose an activity, such as speaking. Go ahead and speak. Notice any misuse, such as a tight throat, forward chin, and so on.*

2. *Now just think about doing the activity, but do not do it, so that you inhibit your immediate response to speak. Continue to notice that your throat wants to tighten to speak, but do not speak.*

3. *Instead of speaking, bring your attention to the top of your spine and the bottoms of your feet as you give yourself the basic directions for suspension and support.*
   - *Allow my neck to be free.*
   - *Allow my head to free forward and up, or away from my spine.*
   - *Allow my back to lengthen and widen.*
   - *Allow my shoulders to widen, and my arms to free out of my back.*
   - *Allow my ribs to move with my breath on my sternum and spine.*
   - *Allow my knees to release forward and away.*
   - *Allow my feet to be on the ground.*

- *Allow the ground to support me.*
- *Allow my ankles, knees, and hips to be open to receive the support.*
- *Allow the support from the ground to come up through my legs, spine, and head.*
- *Allow myself to breathe, and notice the room.*

4. *As you stay with your basic directions, you now have three choices as to what to do next.*
   - *Choice 1: not to do anything as you give your basic directions.*
   - *Choice 2: to do something different from speaking—like lifting your arm, or swinging your leg—while you give basic directions.*
   - *Choice 3: to gain your original end—to speak—as you give your basic directions.*

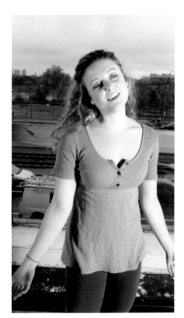
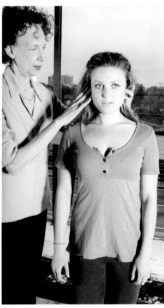
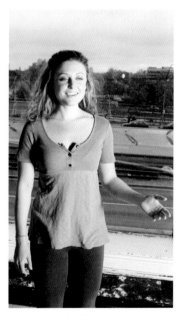

| Speaking with habitual misuse. | Giving basic directions. | Choice 2: lifting your arm with basic directions. |

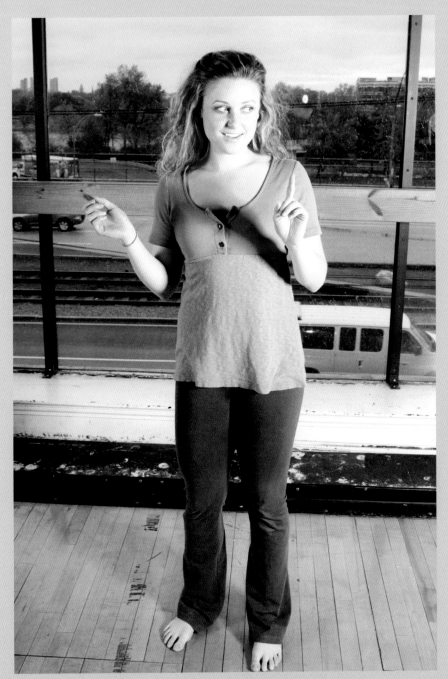

Choice 3: speaking with basic directions.

The idea here is not to go on in the same habitual way. If you feel you cannot stay with your basic directions as you do your original activity, then you can choose to do something simple like raising your arm as you direct. Or you can choose to do nothing but give yourself basic directions until you can stay with your basic directions and speak. This results in you being able to speak with your neck free without tightening your throat.

Do the Three Choices exercise as many times as you like using the same stimulus, "to speak" in our example, and you will find surprising results when you decide to attempt the original activity again. Try this process with sitting, standing, walking, texting, talking on a cell phone, or singing. I also call this exercise "What if I didn't do that?"

While you are working on these exercises, be careful not to tense up your body to prevent yourself from doing too much. Alexander said, "When you are asked not to do something, instead of making the decision not to do it, you try to prevent yourself from doing it. But this only means that you decide to do it, and then use muscle tension to prevent yourself from doing it."[5] In other words, tensing your body so that nothing happens is not the same as stopping the habit.

Each time you say "no" to a habit, it becomes less imprinted on your brain. Each time you do an activity a certain way, a pathway is carved out in your brain. As you do it again and again the same way, that pathway gets deeper and deeper, and other pathways are less available. You must stop using the habitual pathway in order for other pathways to be available. As you use alternative pathways, different from your habitual self, your sense of self changes.

During my first experience with the Alexander Technique, the most interesting moment came when I realized that I felt different. I was still me, but my sense of self had changed. I was not the me that I always knew. I had learned to inhibit many aspects of my habitual self. With awareness, over time, I changed how I thought, how I moved, and how I responded. I became freer.

While we were working on exploring inhibition, an acting student found a way to connect with himself in a new way. After doing the Three Choices exercise to explore inhibition, he found, "I finally understand inhibition. As I did the exercise, I realized that I always pulled my head to one side, and pressed down on my solar plexus before I spoke. I never noticed this before. When I stopped pulling on my head and pressing on my solar plexus, I got hit in the face with my own feelings." He had a very visceral example of inhibition, and what his habits were blocking him from feeling.

In another class, Mary also had the experience of using inhibition to open herself up to her previously unexplored ground. "As I did the Three Choices exercise, I found a habit I never knew I had. Before I spoke I pulled the bottom of my shoulder blades together, and my character's words sounded empty. When I inhibited the pulling in my shoulders, I felt my voice come up like a powerhouse from the ground."

Exercise to Explore Inhibition: Chairs

A very common tendency for an actor is to rush, racing along too fast through the text. Inhibition can be a great help with this. I observed actress Olympia Dukakis give a master class where she taught the following exercise that supports inhibition.

Preparation: *Choose a monologue or piece of text to work with. Place two chairs near you in a cleared space.*

1. *Sitting in one of the chairs, start speaking your text.*
2. *Every time a thought changes, move from one chair to the other. Continue working through the piece, changing chairs each time there is a change in thought in the text.*

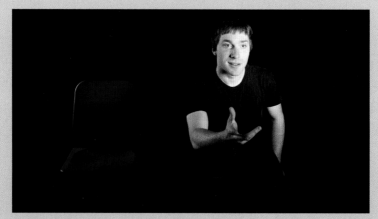

Speaking in the first chair.

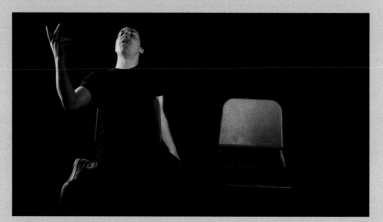

Moving to the second chair as the thought changes.

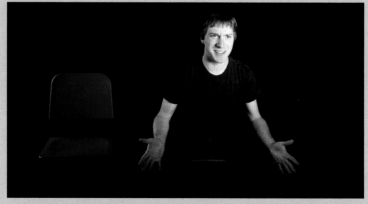

Returning to the first chair as the thought changes again.

This exercise allows for a pause between thoughts, and gives time for the new idea to arise. Most important, the slight pause broadens the depth of feeling in your body, and that depth gives space and time for the idea to expand into your body and voice. While you wouldn't necessarily take this kind of time between thoughts while in performance, or during a take, allowing yourself to explore the text in this way opens up many new possibilities to explore that you can then use for a more nuanced take on what you're saying.

There is bidirectional communication between mind and body. This means that as you have a thought, something happens in your body at the same time. Or if something happens in your body, messages go to your brain. This is especially true in your belly because there are many nerve pathways from your belly to your brain. This accounts for what we call a "gut feeling." Try the Chairs exercise to explore inhibition while noticing what happens in your belly. Do you react habitually, or are you able to stop, inhibit, give basic directions, and respond from a more integrated organization?

Exercise to Explore Inhibition: Nondoing Meditation

People practice many different forms of meditation. Whatever your practice may be, try this exercise as an experiment in finding the moment of inhibition.

Preparation: *You can sit in a cross-legged position either on a chair or on the floor, or sit on a chair with your knees aimed forward and your feet flat on the floor.*

1. *Close your eyes. Let your breath flow easefully in and out.*
2. *Begin to notice your thoughts. When a thought arises, we tend to grab onto it and either try to figure it out, or we let it continue to chatter on and on. Instead, for nondoing meditation, notice that there is a thought but do not respond to it by focusing on it or letting it run wild. Instead, inhibit the habitual response. You don't have to reject the thought*

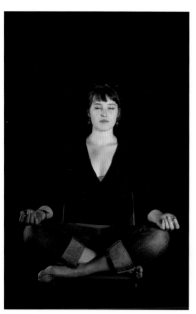

Nondoing Meditation.

and push it away. Neither do you have to welcome the thought and try to sort it out and analyze it. Just let the thought be there without responding to it.

3. *Continue to breathe in and out, and if another thought arises, just let it be. Don't respond to it. You will likely find that your thoughts will start to subside.*

4. *Another way to approach this meditation is to ask the question, "What if I didn't respond to that?" The "that" can be a thought or image coming from within or an outside stimulus, like a phone or doorbell ringing.*

As your thoughts begin to subside, notice what happens in your body. **Inhibition can feel like an absence of something rather than a doing of something.** As you practice this nondoing meditation, you may notice a wave of calmness arise, or an optimal breath with a reflex inhale, or a sigh of relief. Allow yourself to be able to be more present, and experience that calmness and relief that can sometimes come with it.

As you explore the concept of inhibition, ask yourself, how little do I need to do to convey something? You may be surprised to discover that you can do less. If you still find yourself "trying," which is actually a form of endgaining, you may want to stop the trying, because it is the motivation that causes misuse. Instead of "trying," change your intent or desire of what you want. Instead of trying to show that you can "nail the monologue," change your desire and stay present, connect to the circumstances in the life of the character, and act from there. As you explore, you will find it is easier to try something else if you are not focused on fixed concepts.

A few months ago I taught an Alexander Technique class on inhibition. One of the tasks in the class was to write in a notebook, inhibiting your habitual response (such as leaning down or gripping the pen), and to give basic directions in order to write with improved use. One student tells his experience: "Once I completed the activity of writing notes in my notebook with inhibition, Betsy asked me how I felt. I told her that it felt funny rising away (lengthening my back upward) from my notebook, and it became increasingly difficult to continue doing my activity, the writing. It's hard to multitask: writing in my notebook while I 'Alexander' [gave my basic directions], I said.

"Betsy was very interested and became slightly confused. She then went on to say, 'Doing Alexander while you do an activity is about nondoing and not about multitasking. In this case, it's about not pulling down as you write in your notebook. It is being present with basic directions in the activity. It's not doing another activity. Doing Alexander and an activity is not the same as talking on the phone while you cook eggs.' I then realized that my description of doing an activity with Alexander as 'multitasking' was not appropriate. Inhibition was more about doing less and staying present with what is."

This chapter dwells on the inhibitive, or nondoing, aspect of life. Inhibition is a major function of the nervous system, which is at work all the time. Charles Sherrington, who received a Nobel Prize in Physiology and Medicine, discovered that the nervous system is actually made up of inhibitory and excitatory nerve cells.[6] We are inundated with stimuli and information all the time. We could not possibly pay attention to all of it. So the inhibitory function of the nervous system is constantly weeding out what we do not need and saying "No, don't pay attention to that . . . or that . . . or that." What we end up with as a result of nondoing, or inhibiting, we call presence.

CHAPTER 9

Voice

The human voice has the ability to move us like nothing else. John Gielgud's booming voice reciting Shakespeare or Ella Fitzgerald singing a song can bring us to the edge of our seats. The power of the voice can bring us to laughter or to tears and open our hearts. Your physical and vocal presence tell the story from the stage. If an actor has "misuse" or faulty body mechanics, the voice may be held, squeezed, or pushed out, creating excess tension, which is the cause of many vocal disorders. It takes physical work to produce sound, but how much? And when are you causing the body to overwork, leaving muscles fatigued?

The exercises in this book help sort out what can be controlled, what can be left alone, and what can take care of itself when you are using your voice. With the help of the principles presented, you can gain fuller capacity for breath, more connection to the text, increased ease in vocal range, and a stronger sense of presence and support for all vocalization.

Many actors are told to project their voices. However, **sound does not project. It resounds and vibrates, like a bell. Light projects.** This misunderstanding causes many actors to pull down their head and neck unnecessarily and to strain their voices trying to project. To get your voice to carry without excess tension, you must have a connection to the text and a resonant container, or body. You want to connect, not project.

One of my students had been to many voice teachers and vocal coaches. She was told that her voice was thin and small, and that she needed to work hard and push to make her voice stronger. Using this method she got sore throats, jaw tension, and vocal fatigue, and her voice did not get stronger. When she started to work with me, I taught her first to stop—inhibit—all the pushing and pulling. As she was able to allow her neck to be free, allow her head to release forward and up, and allow her back to lengthen and widen, her voice began to open beautifully. She had a sense of support from the ground as her whole body expanded to resonate with her sound. Her voice became stronger with less effort.

Cornelius L. Reid, a master voice teacher, understood the complex components that are involved in training a voice. "By viewing the 'voice' as an extension of the person, it becomes apparent that 'growing up' vocally can be just as trying an experience as growing up physically and emotionally."[1] Your journey to an expanded self includes a quest to find your voice and "grow up" vocally. For many people this includes learning proper use, breathing, and improving sensory motor skills—how you move. This is not always an easy task, especially if there is some history of trauma. The exercises in this chapter take a closer look at how to use the voice and breath mechanism properly for improved use.

Larynx Suspension

Some understanding of the design of the vocal mechanism can be helpful in developing and producing a strong voice that is resonant and full of overtones. Overtones are all the sounds that accompany one specific sound and enrich overall sound.

The body is a suspension system, which means that all the muscles are slightly extended or lengthened for efficient functioning. This lengthening is very important for strong and lasting vocal power. By design, your larynx is suspended by muscles on the top and on the bottom. The muscles support the larynx from front to back. The larynx looks something like an old-fashioned microphone in a recording studio, suspended by wires in front and back, and top and bottom, to hold it up. When the larynx is suspended and undisturbed in this way, it can function properly. One of its functions is to duplicate vibration and sound. When the ear hears a pitch, the larynx is designed to be able to duplicate the vibration of that pitch.

More often than not, the larynx is not in its proper position and is not suspended. When the head is dropped back, it pushes the larynx forward and down, and the larynx is displaced. In this case, when the ear hears a pitch, the displaced larynx is not able to duplicate the vibration of the pitch so easily. Other muscles in the jaw and tongue have to work to create the pitch, which creates a struggle. There is a clamp down in the larynx, while the sound wants to rise up through the throat and larynx. Since the sound has to push up against the clamped-down jaw, the sound becomes labored. This sound will never be pure and full of overtones and will always be pushed. In addition, overusing muscles in this way can cause fatigue and damage to the vocal system.

One actor I worked with had so much tension in his head and jaw during a performance that he ended up with lockjaw and could hardly speak. The resonating cavities in his head were so contracted that they could not produce sound. After doing the following larynx suspension exercise, his jaw released, and his voice changed markedly. He said, "I'm using different resonators in my head, rather than just in my throat and chest. I had often tried to get these higher resonators working but could not. Now that I am using these other resonators, I'm getting more pleasure out of acting than I ever have." You can see here that faulty use can interfere with your artistic choices for portraying a role.

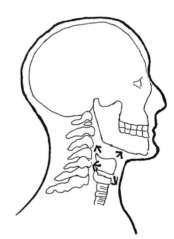

Arrows show the direction of larynx suspension.

Another student I worked with also had an incredibly tight jaw. She had done many exercises and had seen many doctors to try to solve the problem. Nothing had helped her for a deep and lasting change. One day she came in for a lesson and said, "I've finally figured out my jaw problem. When I was young, I went to dancing school, and the teacher always said, 'Smile through everything. When you miss a beat, smile bigger.' I've been smiling through everything since I was four years old. No wonder my jaw is tight."

Exercise to Explore Larynx Suspension

Preparation: *Do the Tracking Your Sensations Exercise to feel the sensations in your whole throat area. Notice if there is any throat tension that arises, and how it affects the rest of your body (the shoulders, the belly).*

1. *Sense your larynx; you can also feel it by putting your hands on either side of the front of your neck. You will probably notice tight muscles around your throat area.*

2. *In the diagram, see the direction of the muscles above and below your larynx that suspend it. See if you can feel the suspension. The larynx can be held or tight for many reasons, many of them emotional. If you find it difficult to feel the suspension, pause here, take some time, and do the Exercise to "Be With" or the Exercise to Explore a Stuck Place.*

3. *To explore the larynx suspension in relationship to your whole body, now stand with your legs apart and your arms open above your head. Feel the diagonal stretch from your right fingertips to your left toes, and from your left fingertips to your right toes. Your body forms an X. The X has you reaching up through your fingertips and down through your feet, creating expansion throughout your body. This expansion supports the suspension in your larynx. Include your expanded field of attention.*

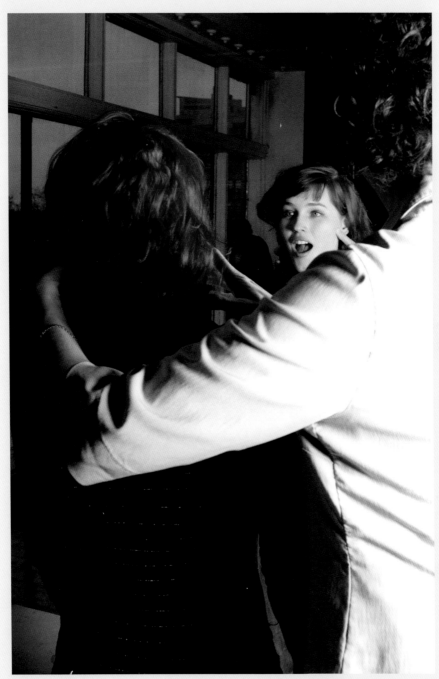

Exploring your larynx.

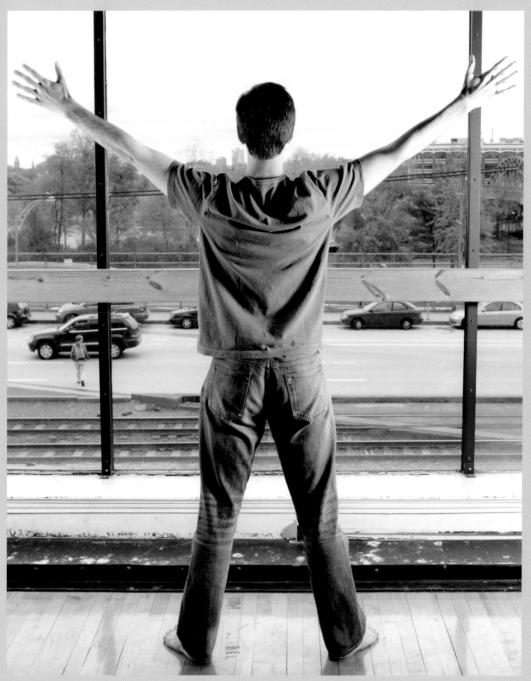

The body forms an X to support larynx suspension.

4. *Vocalize different vowel sounds as you stand this way. Be sure to aim up along your spine as you exhale. Can you maintain the expansion as you vocalize? If not, where do you collapse? What happens in the rest of your body as you vocalize with a suspended larynx? Can you feel the vibrations in your body, ringing like a bell? Can you hear the resonance in your voice?*

5. *Remember that your lungs extend one inch above your collar-bone. Filling this area with air as you breathe supports larynx suspension.*

Losing the suspension in your larynx can have many causes, including any downward pull of your head, or the collapsing of your chest, or even stage fright or anxiety. Reid noted the connection between the suspensory muscles and anxiety: "Chronic muscular contraction within the respiratory tract brought on by anxiety arrests free movement, and this condition seriously impairs the muscular

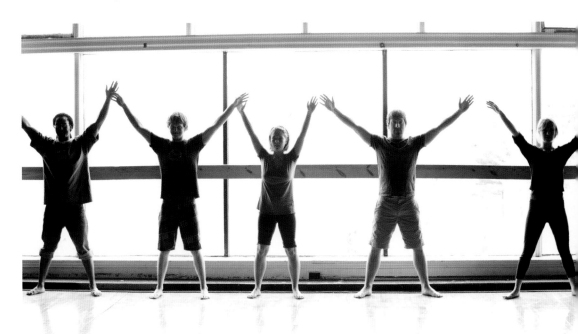

A group practicing the X position to support larynx suspension.

adjustments governing registration as well as the action of the suspensory muscles that position the larynx."[2]

There are deep connections between your voice, your emotions, and who you are. When your body is contracted and pulled down, your voice is too. When you are nervous or anxious, it shows in your voice. The defensive "freeze" response can seriously limit your vocal power, the tightening and contracting interfering with your ability to fully express yourself.

Your Own Voice

Many times students come for lessons and want to improve their vocal power. **However, they want to change their voice without changing themselves.** This will not work effectively for lasting change. The use and overall attitude of your whole being is reflected in your voice. This next exercise lets you take the time and space to be with your own voice and discover some things you might not have noticed before.

Exercise to Explore Your Own Voice

This exercise can be done by yourself or with a group.

1. *Say the following phrase using your name: "My name is _____, and this is my voice."*

2. *Say the phrase again, and add a word that describes your voice. "My name is _____, and this is my voice. My voice is raspy" (or loud, or tired, and so on).*

3. *Give your basic directions for suspension and support, and think about the larynx being suspended and supported. Take your exhale to its complete conclusion, so that you get a reflex inhale.*

4. *Now repeat this phrase again: "My name is _____, and this is my voice." Notice if anything has changed after giving your*

directions. See if there have been any shifts in your voice, body, or being.

5. *Take a few three-dimensional breaths, letting your ribs expand in all directions, and repeat the phrase: "My name is _____, and this is my voice." Do you notice more volume in your voice? More support of the breath and sound?*

6. *Repeat the silent "la la la," letting your breath extend up along your spine as you exhale. Now try saying the same phrase again: "My name is _____, and this is my voice." Do you notice that the longer exhale has an effect on your sound? Is the sound fuller? Does it have more focus? Can you let your voice explore this unknown territory?*

7. *Repeat the phrase: "My name is _____, and this is my voice. My voice is _____." Say a word that describes your voice now, after giving your directions and extending your exhale. You may find your voice has become more booming, stronger, or clearer.*

With this exercise, merely saying the phrase with your own name demands that you connect to the depth of your voice. With this connection you claim the reality of the condition of your voice. You become fully present with your voice, and your self. You can also do this exercise using the phrase, "My name is _____, and this is the depth of my voice."

An actor I taught said, "As I say my own name, it's like a pinball bouncing around in my inner life, touching many aspects of what I'm saying." Saying your name and paying attention to your voice and breath connects you with the present, to your full self.

You may notice that your voice feels shallow and disconnected, or it may be clear and connected. Perhaps your voice can fill the room with your heart, soul, and being. Exploring different kinds of breathing allows you to change the depth and quality of your voice, which can allow your characters to have different qualities and depth to their voices as well.

The Omohyoid Muscle

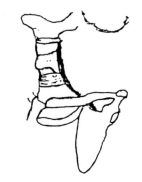

The omohyoid muscle connects the shoulder blade to the hyoid bone, which is above the larynx.

Sometimes vocal problems such as loss of power and control are a direct result of misuse. As we saw in the chapter on use, one very common misuse is lifting your shoulders. This can be particularly harmful to your voice. There is a muscle that connects from your shoulder blade to your hyoid bone, which is above your larynx, called the omohyoid muscle. **When your shoulders are tensing in any manner, this contracts your omohyoid muscle, and your larynx contracts also.** This interferes with the tone, timbre and resonance of your voice. Having an awareness of the omohyoid can help ensure that you are not tensing your larynx.

Exercise to Explore the Omohyoid Muscle

Preparation: *Look at the diagram and see how the omohyoid connects to your shoulder and to your hyoid bone above your larynx.*

1. *Feel the connection between your larynx and your shoulder through the omohyoid muscle.*
2. *If you tense your shoulder at all, your larynx will tense also. Shoulder tension is caused by many misuse habits, including, but not limited to, pulling your head down, overarching your back, or lifting or pulling down your shoulders. Do you feel any shoulder tension? Notice what happens in your whole body because of that tension in your shoulders.*
3. *As you notice the tension in your larynx and shoulders, be with it. Do not try to change it immediately. Bring your awareness to your whole body, find support, and breathe. Allow your neck to be free and your whole back to lengthen and widen. As your shoulders widen, you may notice less pressure in your larynx as it returns to its suspended state.*

4. *Now explore speaking. Choose any piece of text. As you speak, be aware of any tension in your shoulder, and how the tension may affect your larynx.*

One student was able to use this exercise to solve a dilemma involving his voice and shoulder tension. "I realized that I had lost some of my vocal power. My volume, tone, and overall control seemed to be lacking. At the same time, I noticed that I formed a new habit of pulling down and holding tension in my shoulders. I soon discovered through my work with Betsy that the two were connected. I was holding tension in my lower back and arching it, causing my shoulders to tighten. When I directed properly, my vocal range and strength all came back. My voice was now coming from a much lower and visceral place. My work in the play I was rehearsing became easier and more honest."

Tongue Tension

Another very common misuse involving your voice is your tongue. As you can see in the diagram, the tongue is very large and fills your whole jaw. Do you speak and listen by tightening your neck and throat? If you do, there will be some degree of tension in your tongue. When you drop your head back and down as we saw in chapter 3, "Use and Misuse," you displace your larynx forward and down. This forces your tongue and jaw to tighten, causing throat and vocal trouble. When you drop your head back and your jaw tightens, the whole alignment of your mouth is off-balance and can cause temporomandibular joint (TMJ) problems and teeth grinding.

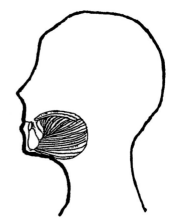

The tongue muscle.

Exercise to Explore Tongue Tension

1. *Put your thumb under your chin and feel what the area feels like without speaking. The muscles should feel soft and mushy, and you should easily be able to push them in toward your jaw.*

2. *Begin to speak, with your thumb under your chin. Notice there is movement there now. Has that soft muscle become hard? Can you still push it in? As you speak, you want that area to remain soft even when your tongue is moving. If your tongue is tight, ask yourself, "Can I do less?"*

3. *Try this exercise with a high-stakes piece of text. If your tongue is forcing pressure down on your thumb, there is too much tension. As you speak again, see if you can lessen the pressure on your thumb to be sure you are not overtensing your tongue. If your head is dropped back and down, your tongue and jaw automatically tense. Allow your head to release forward and up.*

4. *Repeat step three again, and this time combine your understanding of this exercise with the exploration of the omohyoid muscle. When your tongue, larynx, and shoulders are free, your ribs can move for your breathing, and your voice is free and supported to express a dynamic range of character choices.*

When the back of your tongue is tight, it is difficult to connect thought and intention, because the pathway is blocked in your throat. When this happens, your voice gets swallowed from the pulling down in your larynx, and the vocal mechanism has to push up to make sound. Remember that you want a resonant container like a ringing bell. Don't hold your breath and squeeze the back of your throat, tensing your tongue as you speak. Relieving yourself of these excess tensions allows your voice to be free enough so that what you say can come through clearly and truthfully to your fellow actors, and to the audience or camera.

Regarding throat tension, one student spoke about his work with Shakespearean text. "Shakespeare work requires me to live in a highly emotional state for an extended period of time. I would often come away from doing a scene with a headache and a strained throat. Betsy's work was the key I found to maintaining a high-stakes situation without hurting my instrument. Now that I've stopped tightening my larynx while speaking text, I no longer have a sore throat after working on a scene."

The Voice of a Character

When you begin working on a role, you may notice that your character speaks in a voice that is different from yours. How do you make these changes? Many actors overlay a voice that they think is fitting. For example, if someone is playing a young ingenue, a typical choice might be to put on a soft, coy voice with a Southern accent.

My approach to finding the voice of the character is to find his or her breathing first. How might he or she breathe? Would the character have more movement in his or her ribs, or belly, or whole torso? How fast might his or her ribs and belly move, as opposed to yours? What speed might his or her breathing be?

To see how different people have different voices and different use of their breath, choose a partner to work with. Try exploring your partner's voice and breathing. This will give you some idea of just how different breathing patterns can be, and how these breathing patterns create your character's voice for both speaking and singing.

Exercise to Explore the Voice of a Character

This exercise can be done with a partner or a group.

> 1. *Partner A (she) lies down on the floor to work. Partner B (he) sits by her side.*

2. *Partner B watches Partner A's breath move in and out. Pay attention to the way her ribs and belly move—how much, and at what pace. You may also put your hands on your partner's ribs and belly to feel the movement, in addition to seeing it.*

3. *While still sitting by Partner A's side, Partner B takes on Partner A's breathing pattern. Partner B moves his own belly and ribs at the same speed as Partner A, and expanding and contracting his ribs and torso in the same manner as Partner A.*

Partner B, you may discover that your belly moves a lot as you breathe and your partner's belly does not move very much at all, or vice versa. This will affect your whole body and will produce a different voice. When you move your belly and your ribs at a different speed than your partner, you change the timing of your breath, and this transforms your body's whole orientation and visceral experience, and so your voice has a different quality, timbre, and resonance.

4. *Partner B begins to notice changes in himself in body tension, sensation, thinking, and emotion.*

5. *Partner B then stands and walks around the room, moving his body with this new breathing pattern of Partner A. Partner B tries speaking from these changes. Partner B may feel odd when allowing these changes to take place. There may be a different vocal quality, caused by taking on someone else's breathing pattern. The vocal changes that take place come from the breath and visceral changes Partner B has newly embodied, not by "putting on" a new voice.*

6. *If you are in a group, change partners and repeat the whole exercise.*

7. *Now explore finding the breath of a character. Working on your own, imagine what the movement of the character's breathing might be. You probably observed different qualities in your partner; what of these might your character have?*

A Southern ingenue's breathing might be slow, and there may be more motion in her chest and less in her belly. A race-car driver or athlete might have faster breath placed lower in the belly. These different breathing patterns create different vocal patterns. Explore the different possibilities of what your character's breathing might be like.

The Art of Using Verse

George Trevelyan was a student in Alexander's first teacher training course in 1940. He was a poet and an actor and gave many readings. I met him in 1988 at an Alexander Technique International Teacher's Congress in Brighton, England, where he gave a lecture on "The Art of Using Verse."

Trevelyan presented a true Alexander perspective on reciting verse. The elements he discussed included many of the concepts we've been exploring in this book: being present, inhibiting your habitual response, not endgaining, and allowing the unknown to emerge. The exercise below is taken from a handout he provided, and it is reproduced here word for word. Explore this process as an exercise in vocal inhibition.

George Trevelyan's Exercise to Explore the Art of Using Verse

1. *Never learn the words of a poem.*
2. *Get the picture image.*
3. *Listen. Get picture after picture.*
4. *Words give rise to picture—the miracle.*
5. *Speak only a living thought—give consent only to living thought.*
6. *Refuse to say anything that is not a living thought.*
7. *Need to give time to let them [the thoughts] form.*
8. *The words drop into undoing.*

9. *Deliver thought, shut mouth, inhibit desire to go on. Pause between words and phrases. Let lungs fill.*
10. *On the out breath, speak.*
11. *The old way was to suck in air.*
12. *Close lips and inhibit desire to go on.*
13. **When you know there is no need to go on, you can go on.**
14. *Decide to give one more thought.*
15. *Live in thought and stop.*
16. *Take an idea out of the ether and put it in your heart and mind. Act as if it were true—without belief or disbelief.*

Trevelyan recommends that you have a simple thought or image on a single breath. At the same moment, your body will respond to this thought. If you are not able to have an easy, long exhale, do the exercise to explore extending the exhale, the silent "la la la." Then your voice can be free to fill the space all around you especially behind you. Remember your 50-50 awareness and be willing to go into the unknown as you practice this exercise.

Many actors force a booming voice to convey a thought. Instead of sound and fury, try to let a thought simply be there, and then notice that it has a voice. Your body and voice are at the service of the thought. Let your thought drop into your body and voice. That way, the thought, breath, and words are all in sync.

Learning how to relieve vocal tension and explore different breathing patterns helps you know your own instrument better, and allows you to create nuanced and grounded characters. Using these exercises can help you train your voice to be connected to your breath, thoughts, and body. When you can practice this connection—all elements working in sync—and inhibit your habitual reactions, you can have a voice that conveys the specificity of each present moment.

CHAPTER 10
Character and Role

The first character that you develop is your self. We are all born without habitual patterns. We started out in a state of being rather than doing. You can see this with a newborn, just taking in life as it comes. As we grow and life situations arise, we respond and create patterns of thought, movement, and behavior that define our personality, our use.

As an actor, you play many personalities. When you are given a script, you read it while thinking about the story you will tell and what role you will play in that story. You wonder what it would be like to play a character like that: a lover, a killer, a con man, or a saint. You think about how that character's personality is like yours or not like yours. To understand another character, it makes sense for you first to understand your own.

Your Identifications

I call "identifications" any pattern of behavior, personality, or movement that you identify with. Identifications exist on many levels, including mental, physical, and emotional. Habitual identity patterns include "I'm not good enough," "I'm always the victim," or "I'm always right." In some cases, they are physical identifications, such as "I want to feel powerful" or "I need to look sexy."

Here's an example of what I call an identification: As a baby, if you are hungry, you cry to get your mother's attention. But if your mother is busy and unable to feed you, you cry more for her attention. Then, after you cry, she feeds you. A pattern is created. When you want something, you cry. This behavior seems to work.

So you continue to cry when you want something. An emotional identification may be "I am not good enough." This might be from when your parents told you again and again that a neighbor's child gets better grades than you.

Another common identification is smiling, even when it's not genuine. As a child you smile so that your family thinks you are happy. With this, it seems like everything is fine, so everyone can be comfortable. Years later you still may have this kind of fake smile on all the time as a long-held habit, even when things are not fine. Or, if you sprain your ankle when you are four years old, even years down the line you may favor one leg more than the other and walk with a limp. Most people who've had a foot or leg injury still slightly favor one leg or still slightly limp years later. Physically leaning forward is also a common identification. People tend to lean forward to show that they are listening, so that their friends think they care about what they are saying.

All these behaviors, habits, and movement patterns that make up your history build your own character. Alexander advised his students to look at all their habits and beliefs and suggested that they would discover that eighty percent of their habits were not truly formed by their own ideas or beliefs. The habits and beliefs were learned or imposed by others: by family and by religious, social, and work groups.

A student in one of my classes who was brought up in a very polite and well-behaved family was led to believe that it was not appropriate to talk back to an authority figure, even if she had something valuable to contribute to the conversation. Because of this upbringing, she rarely shared her opinions or creative thoughts in class or in rehearsal. Another student with a history of trauma was led to believe that screaming was the only way to win an argument. As she raised her voice in reaction to the smallest disagreement, she lost her ability to reason. The research of trauma expert Bessel van der Kolk has shown that in the moment of an overwhelming incident, the lower reptilian brain takes over for survival while the neocortex, the thinking brain, shuts down. When this happens, it disables you from being able to think and act clearly in the present moment.

Exercise to Explore Your Identifications

Preparation: *Think of one habitual identification or identity pattern you have. For example, "I always feel wrong," "Nobody likes me," "I need to do everything myself," "Nobody is as talented as me." You will find that many of these identifications arise, both positive and negative.*

1. *Begin to name and unravel your personality's habitual identifications or identity patterns. (We'll use the case "I always feel wrong.")*

2. *Notice how often you respond from this place. (I don't speak up in rehearsal if I have an idea about how to play a scene because I think I'm wrong.)*

3. *Notice how it feels in your body.* **Identity patterns have corresponding muscular contractive patterns.** *(When I'm wrong, my body feels stuck, tight, and small, and I feel unable to express myself fully.)*

4. *For an actor it's helpful to be aware of this identification pattern. If your character "always feels wrong," that should be a choice, not your personal identification. If it's not an appropriate identification for your character, you can inhibit your own mannerisms and behavior that make you feel wrong in order to access the truth of that character, which is different from yourself.*

5. *Or, if your character does have this tendency (to always feel wrong), you can recognize your own habits around this and use them. This is where your character meets your self. For example: when you feel wrong, you feel tight and small.*

Exaggerate it or elaborate on it. Consciously feel more stuck. Then bring this feeling to your character, to help you fully experience the character's sense of feeling wrong.

6. *You can also explore the phrase from the Nondoing Meditation exercise to explore inhibition: "What if I didn't respond to that?" For example, if you are feeling wrong about something, can you try feeling wrong but not judging yourself about it?*

Understanding your own identification patterns is an important aspect of your journey to an expanded self. As you are aware of patterns, you can choose to change them. Not "always feeling wrong" opens many other possibilities of thinking and behavior for you. You can ask the question from the Three Choices exercise to explore inhibition: "What if I didn't do that (always feel wrong)?"

After doing this exercise, one actor realized that she was afraid of her own power. She felt this showed up as a tendency to hold back her powerful voice and her body. Her body tended to be contracted and small. Her habit showed up in every role that she played. She wanted to be cast as a leading lady, but no director trusted that she could do it. As she became aware of the pattern, she was able to take steps to change. She did a lot of the Tracking Your Sensations Exercise to find where the contractions were lodged in her body. She used her basic directions and the Counting Exercise to explore breath and sound to get her full stature. And eventually, she did get cast in a lead role.

A Character's Walk

Many habits are hard to change. Walking seems to be one of the hardest, probably because it's something we do so often. It is not uncommon to identify a friend in the distance solely by their walk. For an actor, you must be able to change your own walk so that you are able to transform and walk like your character. If you do not have the accurate walk of a character, you may end up making large gestures elsewhere to convey personality traits to try to convince the audience of who the character is. However, when you have successfully taken on your character's walk, you can do fewer of these big gestures.

Exercise to Explore a Character's Walk

This exercise can be done with two or more people.

Preparation: *Find a room that has enough space to walk around in.*

Part 1:

1. *Walk around the room. As you walk, watch one another, and as a group, name the general components that you see of other people's walk, and of your own. Examples:*
   - *How you set yourself to begin to walk*
   - *Angle of the head*
   - *Shoulder movement*
   - *Length and speed of arm swing*
   - *Back curve*
   - *Hip movement, or lack thereof*
   - *How the knees bend*
   - *Overall freedom of movement*
   - *How and where the foot hits the ground*
   - *What is leading the body: head, knees, or chest*
   - *Speed of the walk*
   - *Sound of the walk*

2. *Name and then write down three of these components that distinguish your walk. A component of your walk that you do all the time is called a habit, like swinging your arms a certain way, or jutting your hips forward. Notice the power of the habit.*

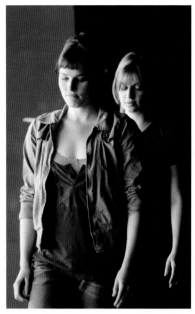

Exchanging walk with a partner.

3. *Pair up with a partner and exchange walks. Take on your partner's walk, and have your partner take on yours. Start by walking behind your partner to pick up components of his or her walk. Perhaps he bangs his foot into the floor, or drops his head forward. After you get the overall feel of your partner's walk, let your partner step aside as you continue to walk your partner's walk. Let your partner watch you.*

4. *Change roles and observe your partner walking your walk. Afterward, check—did your partner emphasize the same components of your walk as you wrote down? The point of this exercise is not to imitate well. It is to be able to recognize, inhibit, and choose to be in or out of your own habits.*

Part 2:

Preparation: *Choose a character. Walk as you recite a piece of text as your character. Then walk and recite the same piece of text as yourself.*

1. *Begin to move around the room as this chosen character.*

2. *Find your character's walk. Write down three components (makes big arm swings, stiffens legs, walks quickly).*

3. *Explore going from your habitual walk (walk as yourself) to your character's walk (walk as the character). How are they different? How are they the same?* **Where does the character meet the self as you walk?** *For example, "We both stiffen our legs," "The character swings his or her arms more than I do," and so on.*

Part 3:

1. *Give basic directions: Allow your neck to be free, allow your head to free away from your spine, allow your back to lengthen and widen, and allow the ground to support you.*
2. *Explore going from your directed walk to your character's walk.*
3. *Is there a difference between going from your habitual walk to your character's walk and going from your directed walk to your character's walk? Name the differences. When you go from your habitual walk to your character's walk, you take your habits to the character. When you go from your directed walk to your character's walk, you approach it from a more spontaneous place.*

Many students have noticed more clarity and focus moving from a directed walk into a character walk. For example: your habitual walk may include jutting your head forward, but your character may not do this. As you give your basic directions for your neck to be free, you are more able to inhibit the habit of jutting your head forward.

Part 4:

1. *Set yourself up for lying-down work.*
2. *Feel the results of what you have been doing—walking. How do you feel after walking? Are any parts of your body tired?*
3. *Think about walking, but don't walk: inhibit the walk.*
4. *Notice the habits in your legs as you think about walking. Try letting them go.*
5. *Think of walking, but don't do it, and then notice the habits in your arms. Let them go.*
6. *Think of walking, but don't do it, and notice the habits in your head, neck, and back. Let them go.*
7. *Notice yourself without your walking patterns. The absence of. . . . You may feel empty of something in one way and full of something else, perhaps other aspects of yourself.*

8. *After this lying-down work, when you are back on your feet, notice where you land after all this attention to walking. Notice how you feel.*

Regarding habitual walking, a student of mine recalled, "I could not seem to change my distinctive habitual walk. After working together for a few minutes, Betsy said that the back of my head was tilting down a bit. When I was able to change the direction of the tilt, I was able to move more freely and change my walk to suit the character I was working on."

A Character's Breath

We have explored breath in chapter 6, "Breathing," and in chapter 9, "Voice." Now we will see that people with different identifications breathe in different patterns. You will see how your breath is different from your character's. The breath of your character distinguishes and identifies your character. An anxious character will often breathe with quicker, shorter breaths. A more relaxed character will have longer, more flowing breaths.

Exercise to Explore a Character's Breath

This exercise can be done by yourself or with a partner.

Preparation: *Lie on the floor on a carpet or a mat.*

1. *Do the Exercise to Explore Optimal Breath with a Reflex Inhale, allowing your ribs to move on your sternum in front and on your spine in back. Allow your belly and ribs to expand as you breathe in, and release as you breathe out. Aim up along your spine as you exhale completely for a reflex inhale.*
2. *Begin to think about your character, and notice how your breathing changes.*

3. *How is the rest of your body affected by this change in your breath?*

4. *Explore your ribs, belly, and breath versus the character's. How are they different? How are they the same?*

5. *What does your character want to do? Notice your breath. Let the character's desire or objective bring you to your feet.*

6. *As that desire gets the character to his or her feet, notice your breath. Try not to have a preconceived "set" as you move.*

7. *To whom does he or she want to speak? Notice your breath.*

8. *What does he or she want? Don't endgain, or do too much to get it. Just think about it and notice your breath.*

9. *What is in the way? Notice your breath.*

10. *If you have a partner, speak to your partner using some of your character's text. If you are by yourself, imagine a partner. Then stop and watch your breath.*

11. *Begin to speak again. Then stop and give basic directions before you speak.*

12. *Does your breath change when you are surprised by what your partner, real or imagined, said?*

13. *Drop the character, walk around the room, and notice your own breath. Do you notice any changes? If it was a high-stakes situation, you may need some time to let your nervous system calm down and self-regulate. Let the ground support you, and begin to look around the room. Do the "describe the details" portion of the Exercise to Explore Presence to bring you to the present moment.*

When you are able to monitor the changes in your breath in the present moment, you begin to understand that many changes take place from moment to moment. If you are holding on to your habitual pattern of breathing, it is difficult for these changes to occur. As you allow your breath to freely adapt to the ever-changing circumstances of a scene or play, you may feel involved and committed to the character and the story in a new way.

One student reported, "After I did the exercise, I understood the character's breath. I felt clearer in my body. I knew where the text lived." When he was able to feel his character's breath in his body, he was able to sense what his character wanted, and he was able to speak the words of the text from his body.

A Character's Thinking, Feeling, and Sensation

We have what is known as a triune brain, meaning that it has three parts. The most primitive and lowest part in physical placement in the brain is the reptilian or instinctual brain. This handles our autonomic systems and survival mechanisms, and it communicates via sensation. The next highest part in placement and evolution is the limbic brain. This handles our emotions and communicates with feelings. The highest part of the brain in placement and evolution is the neocortex. This part monitors our cognitive abilities and communicates via thinking.

Normally the different parts of the brain are used in different situations and different moments in life. When you need to figure out a math problem, you use your neocortex for thinking; when you encounter a fearful situation, you use your reptilian brain. Also, most personalities tend to have a bias toward one part of the brain or another—some people tend to feel a lot while others tend to think and analyze. It is valuable to consciously explore what it is like to be led by these different manners of motivation for communication.

Exercise to Explore a Character's Thinking, Feeling, and Sensation

Preparation: *Choose a character in a particular situation or scene. For example: "I'm preparing a meal for my new mother-in-law," or "I'm going to run away from home." For the exercise we will use the example "I am a young boy and I just met a lovely young girl who I think is the girl of my dreams."*

1. *Say a few lines from a scene, letting the character be driven by thought. ("I keep thinking how wonderful it will be to grow up and get married and raise a family with her.") Let thought after thought arise and lead you through the scene.*

2. *Now try the scene with the character driven by feeling. ("I feel so happy. I feel so excited about meeting her.") Let emotion after emotion arise as you explore the scene.*

3. *Go through the scene now with the character driven by sensation. ("I feel my heart beating fast, my legs feel weak.") Allow the sensations of the character to flow as you act the scene. Notice one sensation after another. They can be small shifts that we often do not notice, like trembling or buzzing.*

4. *Take some time and notice the difference between these three different modes of driving through a scene.*

5. *Now give yourself basic directions for suspension and support. Repeat the exercise and direct before each time you do the scene initiating from a different part of the brain:*

6. *Direct and do the scene with the character driven by thought.*

7. *Direct and do the scene with the character driven by feeling.*

8. *Direct and do the scene with the character driven by sensation.*

What was the difference between steps 1, 2, and 3? Which step gave you a more realistic performance? What happened when you added directions? Did you feel more present with your scene?

One young man was playing an accountant in a show. His character thought about numbers all the time. As he did the scene driven by sensation, he said, "I felt the numbers on the skin of my arms." Another student remembered her experience of the Three Choices exercise to explore inhibition. She remembered that as she chose to inhibit to speak, she always began to think first. She realized, "As I prepare to speak for any character I play, I noticed that I push all my energy up to my brain to think about it. I never let my sensations speak. What if I didn't do that? I would have the most amazing potential available to me."

Exercise to Explore Approach to Character and Script

The script is the written text that you will speak. A script may be loosely written, leaving you room for improvisation, or it may have dialogue that is intended to be spoken word for word. Either way, you want to understand how to approach the script. If you can, try this exercise before the first time you read the full script.

1. *Track your sensations in your body and make sure that you are aware of your legs and feet. Try doing the Exercise to Explore Support before you read the play. As you read, don't try or work to get something. Let the play come to you.*

2. *As you identify the similarities and differences between yourself and your character, ask: Is the character separate from you? Do you leave yourself to become the character? Do you diminish yourself to become the character? Can you inhibit that contraction and open to the character? As you take on a character, don't contract your body, to separate yourself, so you can become this other person. Find where your character meets you. One student said that before he did the exercises in this chapter, he saw a character as something that lived outside of himself, and something he needed to go to and try to grasp.*

Now he said, "I have myself and I take the character into me, or I go into the character, no grasping."

3. Read the play and hear the story of the play. At first, don't analyze the script. Encounter the script. When you read the play silently and out loud, don't decide what it means. Let the meaning emerge. Ideas about the character will present themselves whether you move into the character or the character comes into you.

4. As you develop a character, never separate your intellect from your body. Do not learn the lines and then teach your body what movement goes with them. As you are learning lines, the lines will come out in a similar manner as how they go in. For example, if you are tense learning your lines, you may be tense reciting them. If your intellect is paying attention but the rest of your body is not, that is a problem and you will need to add body movements later. The reverse is also true. If you learn lines only to certain movements, you'll only be able to do those movements when you recite the lines.

Sometimes the case may be that the director wants you to come in with your lines memorized for a stage play, or you're doing an on-camera scene and have to shoot the scene with barely any rehearsal. For this you need to spend time on you own getting to know your character's breath, movement, use, and voice. You can try learning lines lying down to minimize your habitual movement habits.

5. As you and the director are exploring a character in rehearsal, the director may be in charge of putting together the whole production, but remember that you as the actor have the opportunity to explore and discover the character, with the help and guidance of the director.

6. From the start, the director needs to keep the actors present and keep them not "doing" a preset idea of a character so

that the role can evolve. Be fully available and present with awakened senses, directions in your body, especially in your legs, so that you are grounded and connected to the floor and have an awareness of the room. If that is not happening, the play and the character cannot enter the whole actor. Make room to allow the play to come through. Don't decide to move a certain way. Let decisions be spontaneous, and with inhibition. You need to be present because you do not know what will happen in any given moment.

To play a whole character, understand what he or she thinks, feels, and senses. You embody his or her breathing, movement, and identifications. A character tells a story for a reason. Something in you is related to that reason. In the Exercise to Explore a Character's Walk, we asked the question, "Where does the character meet the self?" It is often the case that there is quite a bit of yourself in the characters that you play—in your movements, emotions, sensations, or thoughts. Discover where your character meets your self as part of the development of the role.

CHAPTER 11
Emotion

The emotional life of an actor must be recognized and cared for. Taking on the life of another demands a very specific ability. You need to be able both to completely understand and to embody another character, and also to be able to lose yourself in the character. If you are not careful, your own emotions can get confused and overextended. You must take care of your own emotional well-being.

There are many ways to do this. Some actors need to make sure that they have some time alone to relax and decompress after a show or a shoot. Others will find it helpful to talk to a close friend or a health care professional. Others may need to take medication, either herbal or allopathic. Yoga, meditation, and breathing exercises also help calm the nerves and heightened emotions that might arise.

It is helpful to do the warm-up and breathing exercises in this book as you take on a character. When you begin from this directed and supported state, you are clear about your own emotional state, and you can therefore separate your emotions from that of the character. Then you can either use your emotions or not, but consciously make the decision.

Common actor patterns of misuse when dealing with heightened emotions can be tense legs, head pulled back, chin jutting forward, breath held, or shoulders braced—all the things that signify "emoting," which is obviously not recommended.

The emotional life of the character must be believable. The body, breath, and voice must convey this accurately. **Many actors make emotional appointments.** For example, someone might decide that when their scene partner says, "I do not love you anymore," he or she has a plan that they will cry at that moment. With emotional appointments, you do not have to be open and vulnerable in the present moment. You do not really have to feel much of anything.

Genuine emotion arises when you are moved or touched inside. Then you have feelings, and they pass through you. *Emotion* literally means "to move through." Feelings are not always comfortable. Often we do not like to feel emotions, but once we feel them, they are acknowledged and can then move through us.

The deeper you block your emotions, the more you might have to compromise elsewhere. One easy way to avoid feeling emotions is to hold your breath. For example, if you feel sad but do not want to cry, you can hold your breath to block the tears. But holding your breath may then become a habit. This habit may interfere with other elements in your life like your health, or speaking, or singing. As an actor you can learn to tolerate strong emotions and communicate a full range of available emotions. The explorations in this book can give you a larger container to hold larger emotions and a larger breath. That way you will not get knocked out of sorts when you have to play big emotions in a scene.

One young woman came in and said, "Since working on the play I've been rehearsing, I was spending half of my days holding back my tears. I have been this way for about two weeks, since I started rehearsal. The more I would ignore it, the more tension came out of it. But when I finally took the time to explore the feeling of being on the verge of tears, rather than ignoring it, I felt like the back of my tongue was closing off my throat, and what I would describe as something like a big metallic rock-balloon would just stay there in the back of my throat all day. I think it also caused me to hold my breath, making my chest and middle back tight. When I focused on the sensation, and allowed myself to feel it and embrace it rather than running away, the rock-balloon got a little smaller. It felt like these little pebbles were sliding down my throat and just falling into my solar plexus. It was such a relief that I couldn't help but smile. My throat tension got progressively less and my breath fell down to my stomach. It was the first time I actively tried to do something about the problem of being on the verge of tears, rather than beating myself up or feeling sorry for myself for feeling this way." She had a very visceral, overwhelming emotional experience, but when she allowed herself to be with the emotion, and give it a shape, feeling, and sensation, the tightness was able to loosen up a bit, and she could get back to really being in the present moment.

Emotion is a big subject. Emotions that are not dealt with can continue to drain your attention and energy, as we saw in chapter 7, "Trauma." Incomplete defensive responses can leave you with physical and emotional stuck places. We also saw that breathing can be very involved in your emotions, especially the habit of holding the breath to not feel unpleasant emotions. A situation of a nagging emotion can be like a tongue on a loose tooth. You are always checking it. It is in the background, but definitely requiring your attention. You are always feeling what is going on. The best and safest way to explore emotion is in a specific and directed way, through the body, the breath, and the mind.

Exercise to Explore Emotion and Body: Your Bubble

This exercise can be done by yourself or with a group.

Preparation: *Find a room that has space to walk around.*

1. *Stand and give your basic directions for suspension and support in your body. Feel the directions extend out to your skin.*
2. *Allow the directions to expand beyond your skin, radiating out of your body, all around you. Your body energy expands to the space around you. This creates a kind of energetic bubble around you. This is one physical component of your journey to an expanded self.*
3. *Walk around with your bubble, your energy field, surrounding you.*

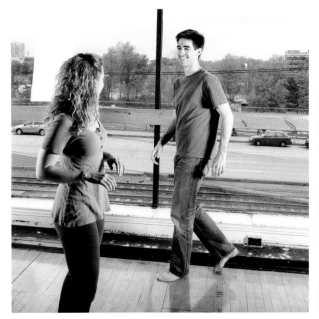 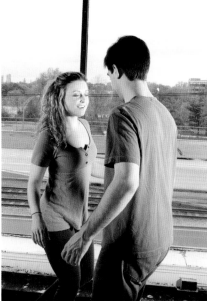

Exploring your bubble at a distance.   Exploring your bubble close together.

4. *As you pass someone, notice if your bubble diminishes, expands, or stays the same. Notice the emotion that accompanies this.*

5. *When you encounter someone else now, practice staying in your bubble. Try this also when you are out on the street, or on the subway. Can you stay in your own space, your own bubble, and not get affected by other people's energy fields?*

6. *Explore what kind of bubble different characters might have.*

Your body emits an energetic force around you. When two energetic forces, two people, come in contact, there is some interaction in these energy fields. For example, you often know without looking that someone is walking behind you as you explored in the Exercise to Explore Boundaries. You can feel their energy bubble. Or you may feel emotionally comfortable in the presence of some people, but not around others.

This exercise begins to bring conscious awareness to the emotions that arise as you become aware of what you are doing with yourself in relationship to another person. It is a common habit to make yourself smaller in the presence of someone you perceive to be more powerful than you (there is an exercise to explore this later in the book). As you explore what it feels like to have the basic directions expand beyond your skin, you can choose your own way of being present when you are alone, or when you are near others.

Emotion and Breath

Think about your own pattern of breathing and emotion. When all is well emotionally, your breath can be full, long, and easily flow in and out. When you are nervous or anxious, your breath tends to be shallow, quick, and labored. **How do you interfere or stop your breathing to control your emotional state?** *Is there an emotion that stops you from being present to explore in the rehearsal room? How does that manifest in your breath and body?*

As we looked at in chapter 6, "Breathing," holding your breath blocks feelings in many ways. The habit of smoking involves a type of holding your breath after you inhale. I have actually noticed that when some of my students have stopped smoking, they realized that they are more aware of feeling their feelings. This isn't a judgment if you do smoke, just an observation about holding your breath in regard to feeling emotions.

Exercise to Explore Emotion and Breath

This exercise can be done by yourself or with a partner.

Preparation: *What emotion is front and center for you? For your character? Notice your emotional state and how you are breathing.*

1. *Speak one minute of text from the script either with a partner or alone.*

2. *Set yourself up for lying-down work with a book under your head and your knees bent, feet flat on the floor. Begin practicing your optimal breath with a reflex inhale, allowing your ribs and belly to move, as you aim up along your spine to exhale. Make sure you take your exhale to its complete conclusion.*

3. *As you breathe in, imagine the breath coming in through the top of your nose and not your nostrils, and allow your breath to touch the top of your spine. This allows the back of your throat to open and your tongue to be released, so you are not suppressing emotion. Because the top of your spine has close neurological connections to your eyes, ears, and voice, this manner of breathing may also help connect your breath to your seeing, hearing, and speaking.*

4. *Do a silent "la la la" as you exhale. Breathe in through the top of your nose. This is a preparation to communicate and to speak with true emotion. Allow your eyes to twinkle. Repeat this step a few times.*

5. *Now, when you get halfway through the silent "la la la," begin to vocalize on the "la la la," almost singing the notes. Repeat this a few times.*

6. *As you exhale, notice the movement in your chest. Is your chest stiff and held, or is it soft and poised? How does this affect your heart? You have the potential to feel many emotions in your chest. But if your chest is held and constricted, you block these feelings.*

7. *With your thumb, feel under your chin to check to make sure that the root of your tongue does not tighten as you breathe in and out. Holding your tongue also blocks emotion.*

8. *Continue breathing in through the top of your nose. Try feeling that emotions can come out of your eyes.*

9. *As you feel your soft palate, allow your eyes to sparkle with emotion.*

10. *Give your basic directions and aim up along your spine so you do not pull down as you breathe.*
11. *Do your piece of text from step 1 with the openness at the top of your nose and the desire to communicate, letting the emotions flow through the text.*

As you practice this exercise, choose to allow yourself to be open to the emotions that arise. As an actor you convey emotion with your frame of mind and your breath. Allow the emotional state of the character to transform your body. Pay attention to your eyes so that they don't glaze over. They are engaged, and you are seeing the world through the emotion. Breathing into your top nostrils keeps your eyes alive and responding to what they are taking in. The expression in your eyes shows the emotional choice you are making.

Many actors in performance get very wrapped up in how they feel, and they can get overly self-involved. One student said to his scene partner in a fit of anger, "I love that you feel things, but I'm more interested in what you make me feel." Obviously you do not want to be so wrapped up in yourself that you ignore your scene partner's feelings. Use your whole body, mind, and spirit to convey the story to others, and be open to what others are giving you. Put your humanity into the character.

Emotion and Thought

As we have seen, every thought you have is reflected simultaneously in your body. A certain emotion makes you feel a certain way. When you are angry, your thoughts and your body reflect the anger, often with tight muscles. When you are happy, you often feel a lightness in your body.

Exercise to Explore Emotion and Thought

This exercise is done with a partner.

Preparation: *Do a scene with your partner. Notice your use. Notice your own emotional needs versus the character's emotional needs.*

1. *Sit across from your partner in chairs or on the floor.*
2. *Partner A: Choose an emotion, positive or negative, and think about the emotion as you breathe in and out. Track the sensations in your body. Don't tell your partner the emotion you are choosing.*

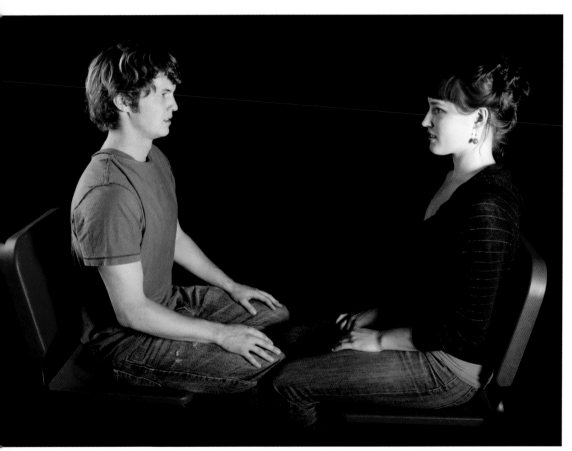

Exploring emotion and thought.

For example, let's look at choosing the emotion of loneliness. Describe how your body feels when you are lonely. How do you use yourself? ("When I am lonely the sensations in my body are compressed.") You may feel things like emptiness or heaviness. Allow the feeling of being lonely to be in every cell of your body, from the soles of your feet to the top of your head, as you breathe. Notice your frame of mind. What happens in your body as you think, "I'm lonely"?

3. *Partner B: Observe Partner A, and now try to name the emotion that Partner A is thinking. Both partners can note how emotion and thought influence breath and body.*
4. *Exchange roles, and repeat the exercise from steps 1–3.*
5. *Now try enacting a scene or monologue, and notice how your thoughts and body convey emotion, and if you're still working with a partner, notice how their emotions affect their body and thoughts.*

As you do this exercise, remember to focus on having emotional specificity and simplicity. Allow yourself to be influenced and touched by what is happening in the scene with subtlety and nuance. As you do your scene, notice that your emotions change from moment to moment. Allow your feelings to move through you. Do not attach to them. It's not about you; it's about the text. Just think the thoughts as you breathe the emotion and see what happens. The capacity for joy and suffering is similar. They are both deep feelings.

As you do this exercise, you can try it with many positive and negative emotions. Positive emotions to explore: love, joy, hope, intimacy, caring, laughter, humor, silliness, optimism, spirit, peace, compassion. Negative emotions to explore: hate, fear, anger, loneliness, helplessness, pessimism, indifference, revenge, anxiety, depression.

You may find that in life you have learned to hold back emotional depth and sensitivity. You may discover that depth and sensitivity can become your strength as you learn to use them. They can become a key into the emotional life of the character. As you learn to become aware of your emotions and how they show up in your body and breath, you can learn to respond to the emotions in the moment. Then you will not need to make emotional appointments.

One student discovered what a powerful effect thought and emotion can have in a scene: Brendan was doing a scene where he was very angry with his partner. After they ran through the scene, which I was observing, I told him that at a certain point, I thought he was going to spit at his partner. He said, "Oh, my God, I totally wanted to spit at him, but I didn't." As he had the thought, breath, and emotional impulse to spit, some muscles in his body were already doing it, which is what I had picked up on. Then when he did not do it, both he and I, the audience member, felt that incomplete action.

There are many more questions to ask about how to deal with your own emotions and the emotional life of the character. To further explore emotions, ask yourself:

- How far do you want to go with emotional thoughts and feelings that frighten you? When you have a lot of impulses and cannot choose what to do, pick the one that is a bit scary and explore it, and flush it out, by tracking the sensations in your body. That way it is not under the surface. You may want to do the Exercise to "Be With" and remember to find your support from the ground.
- What do I do when I get emotionally thrown in rehearsal? Emotional chaos and confusion can turn into artistic food. When something in the text throws you, pay attention to your feelings inside yourself. When a powerful piece of text goes through you, what happens? **Do you choose to react habitually, or do you take a moment to inhibit and respond in the present moment?** You need to step to the precipice every time. It may be agony to express and expose yourself,

but otherwise you are phoning the work in. You are not there in the present.

- How do I repeat a good feeling I had in rehearsal? You do not want to duplicate a feeling by imitating it. You want to create the conditions that produced the feeling. For example: one night in your scene, you felt light and happy because your boss gave you a raise. The next night you may try to duplicate that feeling by reproducing the feeling. Instead, listen to his words, and let your brain think the thought. Your brain then sends messages to your nervous system, your nervous system sends messages to your muscles, and your muscles produce a feeling of lightness. Your body is different. This all happens in a split second.

Our familiar emotional self is enmeshed in our habits. How will these habits change for the character? We have inner emotional templates of who we take ourselves to be. Discover the templates for yourself and your character on your journey to an expanded self. As we see, there are many aspects of an actor's emotional life that need attention. Tending to the use of body, breath, sensations, thought, and the ground for overall well-being is well worth the time and effort.

Part Three
PERFORMANCE

CHAPTER 12

Warm-Ups

Most actors have some kind of routine or warm-up they do to prepare for a performance. These vary from stretching exercises to breathing and vocal routines, running up and down the hallway, or praying for a good show. The warm-up is a very important part of rehearsal and performance. Often, days are emotionally stressful and physically draining. But when it comes time to perform a show at night, how do you get that fight with your boyfriend to stop replaying in your head so you can become your character, who did not have a fight? How do you muster enough energy to perform if you're feeling tired? **How can you use whatever is going on in your life to help rather than hinder your performance?** These next few exercises guide you to come back to a settled place in yourself via tracking, the primary control, inhibition, and direction so that you can begin with fewer habitual sets physically, mentally, and emotionally.

In general, it's a good idea to prepare for a performance or filming a take by connecting to yourself and to your inner instincts, as you bring yourself to the life of the script. You want your muscles to be toned and supple, your breath plentiful, your mind calm, and your voice clear and resonant.

Noticing Your Sensations

As you learned in chapter 7, "Trauma," it is important to be able to track your bodily sensations. When you have an idea of what is going on, you have the ability to change. If you arrive on the set and your nerves are shot from the traffic, address these sensations before you perform. Otherwise they can serve as impediments, preventing your energy from moving and letting you be free to be present in the scene.

Exercise to Track Your Sensations to Help Them Settle

Preparation: *Find a comfortable place to sit in a quiet spot. Keep in mind that the goal here is to explore, not necessarily to relax.*

1. *Begin to turn inward and scan your body. You receive information from your muscles via the kinesthetic sense and from your joints via your proprioceptive sense. Your body and brain support your system's regulation. There is no right way to do this. That would add tension. You can't do it wrong.*
2. *Notice one constriction in your body. (For example, "My throat feels tight.") Notice how that affects the rest of your body.*
3. *Pay attention to your sitting bones. Your sitting bones are an inherent resource. They provide a given support or resting place.*
4. *Gather your awareness and ask, "Where do I feel better?" ("My chest feels fine and my breathing is flowing.")*
5. *Let your whole body integrate the feeling that you feel better. ("There is more expansion in my whole body, including my throat.") See where the change is percolating in your body, and let it spread from there. Now you are ready to continue to warm up your voice and body for a performance.*

You can try this exercise a few different times before you warm up if you are still feeling more than one place of constriction. In step 3, you can use a variety of resources. **A resource can be any thought or image that has a positive influence on your body and mind (your favorite couch, or a memory of a pleasant interaction).** You can also try this after you have finished a performance, to make sure you're letting go of any excess tension that you may have picked up during the course of performing. The directions for suspension and support can be an inherent resource.

An actor in one of my classes had a difficult time just before he walked on stage. He felt like he wanted to hide. He had butterflies in his belly that he was always trying to get rid of. One night, instead of trying to get rid of the nervous feeling in his stomach, he decided to track his sensations. He said, "I stayed with the butterflies and paid attention to my sitting bones, and the butterflies settled like snow in a snow globe. I then gave my directions and got my optimal breath flowing. I felt capable and able to do anything. No trace of wanting to hide." This is a profound shift for just spending a few moments tracking what's happening in your body. Use this as a tool to shift whatever sensations you're feeling that you'd like to shift.

Monkey

One of the major common problems I find with actors is that they do not use their lower body enough. This tends to disconnect the upper and lower body. This is a huge problem because it limits the performance. When you ignore your lower body, you tend to stiffen your legs. Thus you block the impulses that would have you move around the stage. Then you need to convey the story from your head and arms, which is not as complete a performance as you could give if you had access to your whole body connected to the ground. This produces a top-heavy look and does not create believable human and "down to earth" characters. To prepare for acting, start by being connected to the ground. Then you can allow your leg muscles to be less constricted and more fluid and powerful in order to allow the potential for necessary movement. Monkey can help you find this.

Alexander called this exercise "The Position of Mechanical Advantage," because from here, you can move easily in any direction. His students nicknamed it "Monkey" because of what it looks like. Some people today call it "Ready," because you are alert and ready to move in any direction. As you do the Monkey process, you learn to use your legs without interfering with your head-neck-back relationship, your primary control. Also with your legs bent this way, your lower back can widen to allow maximum breath for a resonant voice.

Exercise to Explore Monkey

Preparation: *Stand with your feet hip-width apart. Give the basic directions:*

- *Allow my feet to be on the ground.*
- *Allow the ground to support me.*
- *Allow my ankles, knees, hips, and torso to be open to receive the support.*
- *Allow my neck to be free.*
- *Allow my head to free forward and up, or away from my spine.*
- *Allow my back to lengthen and widen from my hip sockets.*
- *Allow my shoulders to widen, and my arms to free out of my back.*
- *Allow my ribs to move with my breath on my sternum and spine.*
- *Allow my knees to release forward and away.*

1. *As your whole back, including your hips, aims upward, allow your knees to release slightly forward and apart from each other as they bend. Let your ankles, knees, and hips release.*
2. *Renew your basic directions. As your head is leading in a forward and up direction, allow your torso to pivot—not drop—forward from your hips. Keep your weight on your heels. Let your arms hang freely, and allow your shoulders to widen as you breathe.*
3. *Now, to slightly lower yourself in space and get a little closer to the ground, bend your knees. Then pivot forward, aiming out through the top of your head. This position is called a simple Monkey.*

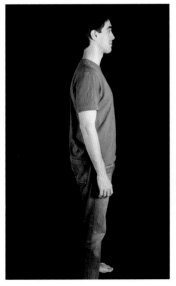
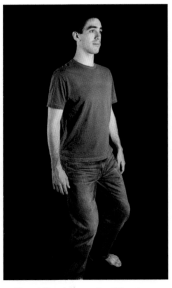
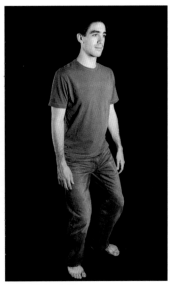

Give basic directions to prepare for Monkey.

Bend the knees for Monkey.

Pivot forward for Monkey.

4. To bend lower, as in the case of picking something up from the ground, continue bending and pivoting for a deeper Monkey.

When you do the Monkey exercise, feel:

- Your head freeing on top of your spine.
- Your whole torso lengthening and widening.
- Your hips moving back and up in relation to your knees going forward.
- Your body weight centered an inch forward of your heel.
- Be careful not to stiffen your legs, clench your toes, or tighten your neck.
- Although Monkey moves downward in space, there is not a pull down in the body.
- When your lower body is free, your upper body can connect and move from your legs.

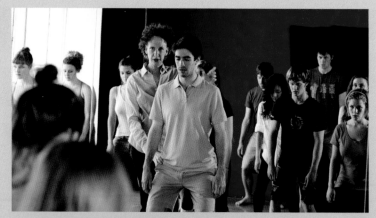

Keep the hips back in Monkey.

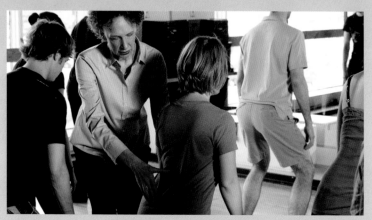

Lengthen the lower back in Monkey.

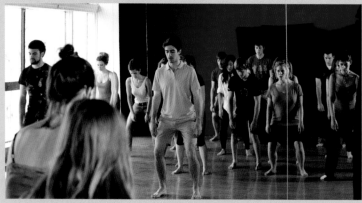

Practicing Monkey in a group.

5. *Try moving from Monkey into different activities. Feel the support from the ground coming up through your legs and torso, and connecting to your arms. Move from that space of grounded support and readiness.*

After learning Monkey, one of my acting students said: "When I did Monkey before a show, I had power in my legs and a connection to the ground that let me go after what I wanted in the scene." Monkey is a simple but powerful exercise that connects you to your whole body as well as to the ground, and it helps you be ready for action.

Hands on the Back of the Chair

The arm joint at your shoulder is designed to be extremely free. It is freer than any other joint in the body—so free that you can dislocate it very easily. But most people do not use it in a way that accesses that freedom. When you reach for something on a high shelf over your head, do you notice that your head and upper back lean back as you lift your arms overhead? This does not access the freedom of the arm joint. Learn to move your arms freely without disturbing your primary control, your head-neck-back relationship. "Hands on the back of the chair" can help you learn this distinction.

Exercise to Explore Hands on the Back of the Chair

Preparation: *Sit in a straight-backed chair and place a second chair in front of you, the seat facing away from you.*

1. *Sit in a chair with your hands resting on your lap.*
2. *Give your basic directions:*
   - *Allow my neck to be free.*
   - *Allow my head to free forward and up, or away from my spine.*

- *Allow my back to lengthen and widen.*
- *Allow my shoulders to widen.*
- *Allow my ribs to move with my breath on my sternum and spine.*
- *Allow my knees to release forward and away.*
- *Allow my feet to be on the ground.*
- *Allow the ground to support me.*

3. *Allow your right shoulder to release, widen, and spread sideways out of your back.*
4. *Allow your right elbow to release out of your shoulder to the side.*
5. *Allow your right hand to release away from your wrist, and your fingers to lengthen out of your hand. Your arm is now stretching out of your back to the side and parallel to the floor. Allow muscles on both the top and bottom of your arm to stretch.*
6. *Gently but firmly, take hold of the top rail of the chair in front of you, with your fingertips pointing to the floor. Continue your three-dimensional breathing and your 50-50 awareness.*
7. *Repeat steps 3–6 using your left arm, keeping your right holding the chair in front of you. As you widen your arms out of your back, this can give you a feeling of opening your chest and heart.*
8. *As you now hold the chair with two hands, open your elbows out to the sides, so that your body can pivot forward. Now try pivoting back, allowing your back to stay wide. Pivot back and forth a few times, as you continue to allow your torso to lengthen and widen.*

The goal is to be able to do this pivoting back-and-forth motion with ease, and without your arms becoming held, heavy, or tense. If your arms get tired, do not stay in this position too long. Drop your

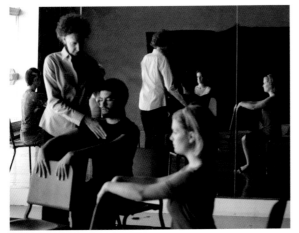

Hands on the Back of the Chair.

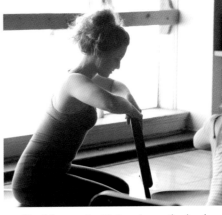

Pivot forward with hands on the back of the chair.

hands to your lap and rest a moment, then do the exercise again. The freedom in your shoulder joint allows your arms to move freely while your head-neck-back relationship is undisturbed. Now you can see that your arms can move separately from your back. Now try lifting your arms over your head without your upper back and head shifting back. **The strength and stability of your back allows the freedom and mobility of your arms.**

One student who tended to have a lot of shoulder tension said, "Actively using 'hands on the back of the chair' in warm-up freed me physically and mentally, and allowed me to see what other tools I could use to bring myself to any rehearsal."

Whispered "Ah"

Walking onto the stage or set is an important moment for an actor. Many actors tend to brace themselves, or hold their breath, or interfere with their breathing one way or another. None of these choices prepare you for a dynamic performance. They may think, "Holding my breath and puffing myself up is a good preparation for walk-

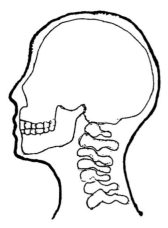

Atlanto-occipital joint and
jaw joint.

ing onto the stage." This can be seen as faulty sensory perception, when what you think you are doing isn't exactly what is happening in reality.

Before stepping on stage, wake up your breath—do not hold your breath. Alexander's whispered "ah" helps you to enliven your breath and prepare your voice to speak. When you walk on stage, you want your breath and voice awake and alive and prepared to communicate in whatever circumstances are arising.

The whispered "ah" is an effective procedure for demonstrating the role of inhibition in breathing and vocal production, and for preparing to speak or sing, making sound without any extra effort. The whispered "ah" also teaches you to distinguish between your jaw joint and your atlanto-occipital joint, which is where your head and spine meet in the center of your head.

Remember that sound is made up of vibrations. A bell rings because of the space inside. The working vibrations create resonance. When your head is freeing away from your spine, your torso can expand. Then there is more space in your torso to resonate with more vibrations.

Exercise to Explore Whispered "Ah"

Preparation: *This exercise can be practiced standing, sitting, or lying down. Follow this set of instructions without pulling your head back and changing the axis of your head. Begin with the basic directions:*

- *Allow my neck to be free.*
- *Allow my head to free forward and up, or away from my spine.*
- *Allow my torso to lengthen and widen.*
- *Allow my shoulders to widen.*
- *Allow my ribs to move with my breath on my sternum and spine.*

- *Allow my knees to release forward and away.*
- *Allow my feet to be on the ground.*
- *Allow the ground to support me.*

1. *Think about something funny and smile to allow the soft palate to go up, thus opening the passages to the throat.*
2. *Allow your tongue to lie on the floor of your mouth and let the tip of the tongue touch your lower teeth. Remember the tongue exploration.*
3. *Let your jaw ease forward and fall down, so that your mouth opens.*
4. *Breathe out with a whispered "ah" sound, as you aim up along your spine. The aim up along your spine is similar to an arrow sitting in a bow and aimed at a target above you. It is poised, alert, and directed.*

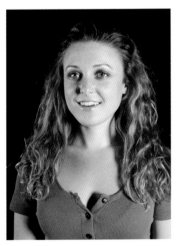
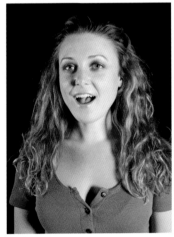
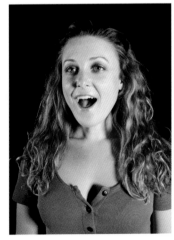

| Smile for whispered "ah." | Mouth opens for whispered "ah." | Breathe out a whispered "ah" sound. |

5. *Close your mouth.*
6. *Allow breath to come in through your nostrils and fill your lungs to the top, which is, remember, one inch above your collarbone.*

7. *Allow your eyes to be alive and twinkle.*
8. *Again, let your jaw ease down, breathing out the whispered "ah." As you try this a few times, notice your breath enlivening your whole system. Can you feel yourself expanding? Notice how you feel in the room.*

When you practice this exercise, focus your attention on each sequential event in turn, and do not allow yourself to jump ahead to make the sound. With attention organized in this way, you can detect and inhibit any unnecessary effort or tension, such as lifting or depressing your chest or sucking in air. As we learned when exploring the optimal breath, when your out breath is full, you get a reflex inhale, your diaphragm naturally springing down and oxygen filling your lungs. This full and easy breath is one of the many benefits you will find as you explore the whispered "ah."

One student I worked with had to shout a lot during the show he was in and was losing his voice after each performance. When he began using the whispered "ah," he said, "The whispered "ah" has become my sword and shield." It became his new way of protecting himself and his voice. This protection allowed him to feel confident and powerful in himself.

Lying-Down Work

The lying-down work is a valuable resource for an actor not only for warm-up and preparation for stage work, but also for health in daily life. When the outer surface muscles can expand and have less constriction, there is more room for the inner visceral organs to expand and deconstrict. This allows more room for movement, which promotes health. We've explored this a little bit in earlier chapters, but here we'll take a closer look.

As an actor, you want to prepare yourself to transform into another character. This often entails becoming aware of, and releasing, your habitual tensions. Then you have a choice to change your use to suit your character. For example, you may tend to overarch your lower back by tightening the muscles there. Perhaps the character you are playing does not. As you do the lying-down work, you can become aware of the overarching in your back and make a choice to let your back muscles lengthen and widen instead. You then walk onto the stage or set with a more believable character and without your personal habitual pattern.

Exercise to Explore Lying-Down Work

Preparation: *Lie down on your back on a carpeted floor or a mat, with a one- or two-inch book supporting your head. Allow your knees to be bent up toward the ceiling, but not pulled together, and allow your feet to be flat on the floor. Allow your hands to rest on your abdomen. Allow the floor to support you.*

Bring your awareness to yourself and notice what is going on inside. Check in with yourself to see if there is any excess tension, if you're holding your breath, or if your mind is racing. Notice what's going on within yourself, but don't try to change anything. Just "be

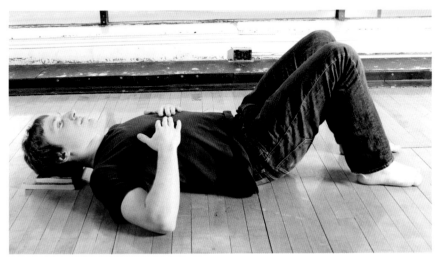

Lying-down work.

with" whatever is going on. **If you try to change yourself by moving or manipulating yourself, you will miss the innate intelligence of your body guiding you.** *You rob your system of its delicate fine-tuning process of self-regulation.*

As you allow the ground to support you, with your eyes open, say out loud or to yourself:

1. *"Allow my neck to be free."*
2. *"Allow my head to release away from my spine or forward and up."*
3. *"Allow my back to lengthen and widen, freeing my muscles, bones, nervous system, and viscera."*
4. *"Allow my knees to aim toward the ceiling so that there is more space in my hip joints and ankle joints."*
5. *"As my ankle releases, my heel drops into the floor and my whole foot spreads out onto the floor, and is not gripping." Repeat steps 1, 2, and 3.*
6. *Now keeping your hands at rest on your belly, continue giving yourself these directions: "Allow my shoulders to release away from my back, my elbows to release away from my shoulders, my wrists to release away from my elbows, and my whole arm to ease out through my fingertips." Repeat steps 1, 2, and 3 again.*
7. *"Allow my hips to lift gently, and then lower back onto the floor. As I lower my hips, allow my lower back to lengthen." Repeat steps 1, 2, and 3.*

As you do the lying-down work, do not try to make things happen. Allow yourself to do less. You are reeducating your system. Keep in mind the principles of inhibition—nondoing and direction. You are not moving yourself around, but allowing micromovements inside. As you are in touch with your primary control and you are releasing into a lengthened state with more space in all your joints, your system will let go of excess tension and free your breathing without you even trying. As you practice the lying-down work, be with your own stillness. Recognize changes. Commit to cultivating them.

Variations of the Lying-Down Work

1. *Do the exercise with inhibition, saying "no" after each direction. For example, say, "Allow my neck to be free." Then say "No, I will not do it in the habitual way." See what happens. You will have a different experience of allowing your neck to be free. Continue, saying "No" to all the primary directions in steps 1–7 above. Prepare not to know what's going to happen, and let yourself be surprised.*
2. *Do the lying-down work with inflatable balls or pillows under your head, shoulders, and hips, as seen in the image.*

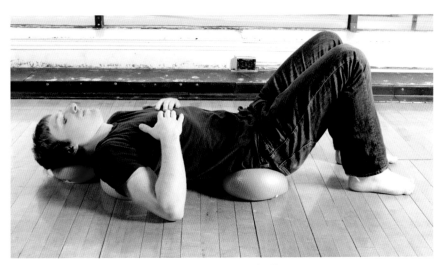

Lying down on inflated pillows.

3. *Do the lying-down work and "be with" what you notice. Inquire to yourself about it, how it feels different or the same. For example: As you bring your attention to your shoulder, you may feel your shoulder pulling in toward the center of*

your body, or downward, or up. Notice the pull. Be with it. Then, ask, "Do I want to pull my shoulder in?" If the answer is yes, continue pulling it in. If the answer is "no," you can stop pulling it in. This is inhibition. This is choice. This is the pathway to an expanded self.

Continue to inquire:

- *Do I need to pull my shoulder in?*
- *What would happen if I didn't pull my shoulder in?*
- *Who is the me that is pulling my shoulder in?*
- *Why would I pull my shoulder in?*
- *What would I be like if I didn't pull my shoulder in?*

These questions give you some choice. When you can notice, be with, and inquire, you can gain a new perspective on long-held habits.

I find when I do my lying-down work that there is an actual chemical change in my body. My nervous system seems to reset itself to a more integrated state. I am more settled and calmer. My orientation is different. I am not endgaining. I feel less anxious. **I feel like I am doing nothing, but that I could actually do anything.**

A student of mine named Jack was struggling with his acting. He said, "I constantly felt the need to use effort in my work. I felt like if I wasn't sweating, crying, and yelling, I wasn't doing anything. I would always do an intense physical warm-up. One day I started exploring lying-down work and giving my directions. It was awesome. It was the first time I felt real ownership of myself. That night at the theater, I started to work up a sweat for my usual warm-up. Then I said, 'Is this really what I need in this moment?' The answer was 'no.' So I grabbed a couple of books and started my lying-down work. I focused on my breath and on my directions. As I lengthened my spine to get up, I felt more open and responsive to stimulus than I ever had been before a show. The show felt great

and natural, without the unnecessary muscle tension that I habitually had in my work."

As you can see from Jack's experience, what you do for a warm-
up is very important. Learn to awaken your whole body, especially
your lower half. Find your connection to the ground, and find your
support. Engage your breath and your voice. You want your thinking and your awareness to be crystal clear as you attend to how
you do what you do. Include your presence, 50-50 awareness, basic
directions, and nondoing (inhibition) for a truly vibrant warm-up
that prepares your expanded self for an engaging performance.

CHAPTER 13

Monologues

Actors often have to speak a long portion of text, or a monologue. This presents many challenges, even to the most seasoned actor. You are on stage or in front of the camera, often alone, and often with a serious dilemma. Perhaps you are deciding if you should kill your wife or not, or whether to tell your boyfriend that you are pregnant. These high-stakes situations are fertile ground for overacting and reverting to your old habits. Try to inhibit these stereotypical responses and allow yourself to go deeper into yourself to find a place of integrity, cohesion, and choice. By doing that you can find balance within yourself, which leads to genuine emotion. This allows you to use an appropriate amount of energy and tension to convey your situation.

Choosing a monologue can be a daunting task for a young actor. Try choosing something that is meaningful for you, and something that helps you learn about yourself. One actor was asked to choose a monologue to work on in a class. He was asked, "What interests you? What might you like to explore?" He said, "I often feel lost and would like to explore that." He chose a monologue that suited that, and began to pay attention to his use and his body. He found that his shoulders were tense and his chest was sinking. His chest felt hollow and empty. He did the Exercise to "Be With" and the Tracking Your Sensations Exercise. As he developed new awareness, he began to understand that the lost, empty feeling was from his past emotional history. Realizing that this was something from the past, he was then able to feel in control and very much connected to his surroundings in the present. Now he had more choices for his monologue. He was no longer bound by the feelings of his past, limiting him only to explore certain feelings and states. His self-inquiry prepared him to be able to have access to a larger range of experiences.

To prepare to work on a monologue, connect to yourself and to the material. As you are exploring this work integrating the Alexander Technique, Breathing Coordination, and Somatic Experiencing with your acting, it is important to remember the acting guidelines for a comprehensive performance. In a master class, stage and screen actor Jason Alexander said there are four basic questions an actor must ask him or herself for the technique of acting:

1. Who are you talking to? Talk to a real person, not an idea.
2. What do you want the person you're talking to to do, and why? What is your objective?
3. What are you going to do to make the other person comply with your objective? What is your specific action or intention? Play a verb.
4. What is in the way? What keeps you from getting it? This is the obstacle.

It is important to find a balance between your acting work (playing objectives, minding blocking) and your inner work (direction, inhibition, and sensory tracking). If you act without your inner work, you rob yourself of subtle connections and choice. If you do your inner work and forget these acting guidelines, you can end up feeling purposeless.

Within yourself, you want to have a clear sense of balance—not only balance of inward and outward attention, but also physical balance. Do you know when you are leaning forward or backward? **A common habit for actors trying to communicate with the audience is to lean forward to convince.** If you are leaning too far forward, there will be excess weight dropping forward. This creates constriction and heaviness, which prevents subtle communication.

Exercise to Explore Finding Balance

Preparation: *Do a one- or two-minute monologue, and notice what is happening with your weight and balance. Are you leaning one way or the other, either front or back, left or right? Does your body feel heavy or light? Notice your tendencies, then continue to the exercise.*

1. *Take a four-legged chair and balance it on two legs.*
2. *Move it forward and backward and feel where the chair feels heavy and where it feels light. You will notice that the chair is heavier when it is closer to the ground and lighter when the chair is upright, closer to balance. When you can balance the chair on its two legs, you will see that it is practically weightless.*

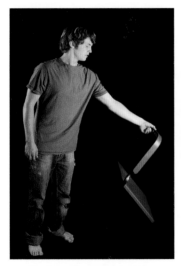 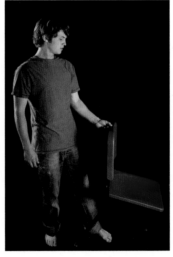 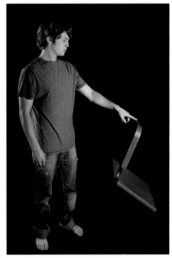

| Explore the weight of the chair forward. | Explore the weight of the chair back. | Explore the weight when the chair is balanced. |

3. *Now do this to yourself. Shift your weight far forward, then far back, and notice the heaviness. Then move less forward, and less back, back and forth, making smaller and smaller movements, until you find that light spot of balance.*

4. *Find a new balance for yourself that feels light and is not pressured down.* **Between forward and back is up.** *This up has potential for subtle, poised, and graceful movement. Your whole body feels slightly lifted, including your heart.*

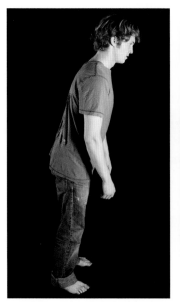

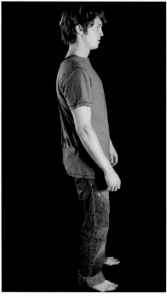

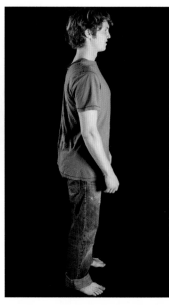

Explore your weight forward.   Explore your weight back.   Explore your weight when you are in balance.

5. *Walk around the room and find the balance and lightness in each step, which is suspension and support in motion.*
6. *Put yourself in any posture or position and explore balance. Try sitting, squatting, stretching, or reaching for something. Move your weight forward and back, and then find the upward balance.*
7. *Now try repeating your monologue again, exploring this new balance. With this new balance, you may have a clearer sense of your bubble, your energetic field.*

I have seen many actors find subtle openings for communication and movement with this exercise. By finding that inner balance, you can express yourself from exactly where you are in yourself. As you learn to find your balance, you will feel less need to lean forward and convince the audience of your objective.

The well-known actress Lynn Redgrave said, "I took Alexander lessons instead of attending movement classes, which helped me enormously in my training and in subsequent years in my acting work. Now I can play people who are graceful and beautiful."[1] I believe the grace and beauty that she speaks of comes from this kind of upright balance.

This efficient exercise is easy to practice as you are standing in the wings waiting to go onstage, or waiting to shoot your scene. It helps you center yourself to better portray the imagined circumstances of your character. **Shift forward, back, up, and go!**

Alexander, Shakespeare, and Crawling

Remember that Alexander developed his technique partially because of his love of Shakespeare. Alexander was losing his voice and was not able to perform. He wanted to be able to continue giving his recitations of Shakespeare's work, so he tried—and succeeded—to solve his dilemma. His love of Shakespeare continued throughout his life. When he had a training course, he had the nonactor participants give a performance of *Merchant of Venice*. Alexander played Shylock in what was said to be a fine performance.

Much of Shakespeare's writing was done in iambic pentameter, a type of meter common in the seventeenth century. **The iambic pentameter pulse is similar to the human heartbeat.** In Sonnet 65, Shakespeare wrote, "Since brass, nor stone, nor earth, nor boundless sea." In this line of text, you can hear the rhythm in the words: bum BUM, bum BUM, bum BUM, bum BUM, bum BUM. When working with iambic pentameter, it is important to get this rhythm into your body. Otherwise there is only cerebral involvement; this can be limiting and not as engaging to watch.

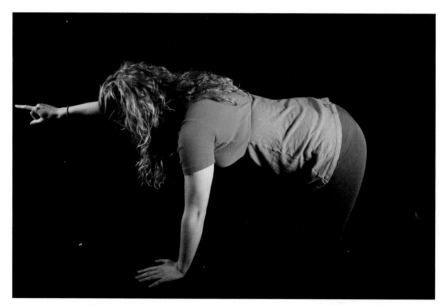

Direction and movement in the same horizontal plane.

Crawling can help you get this heartbeat rhythm into your body. To understand this, look back in evolution, and remember the primary control. In vertebrates—animals with a backbone—the head leads and the body follows in a kind of dynamic opposition. In four-legged animals the direction (up along the spine) and the movement of walking go in the same horizontal plane and in the same path. The direction of the head and back follows the same direction as the line of movement.

But in humans standing on two legs, this changes. The direction, which is up along the spine, is vertical and out through the top of the head. The movement of walking is forward in space and horizontal. In humans the direction and the movement follow different planes.

Crawling gives us the opportunity to experience the direction and movement in one plane or line, like a four-legged animal, with the head leading while the back is following. As you crawl, your right hand touches the ground, then your left knee. This also makes the bum BUM, bum BUM rhythm.

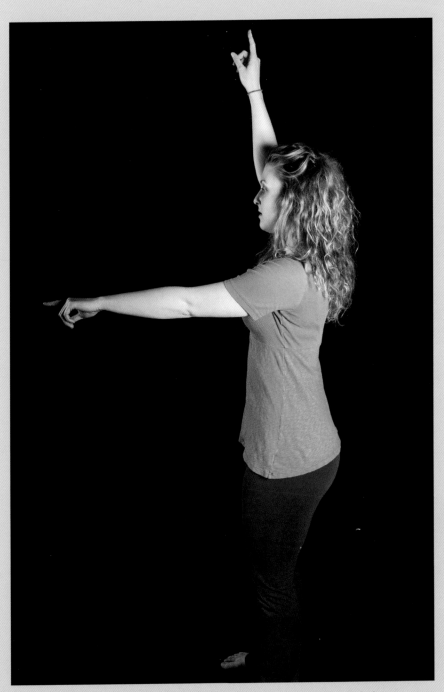

Direction in the vertical plane and movement in the horizontal plane.

Exercise to Explore Alexander Technique, Shakespeare, and Crawling

Preparation: *On a mat or a carpeted floor, place yourself on all fours. Stay here and breathe, and notice how it feels to be on your hands and knees.*

1. *On your hands and knees, palms under your shoulders and knees under your hips, allow the back of your neck to be long. Feel your heartbeat.*

2. *Continue to extend your head forward into space and allow your limbs to follow. Crawling forward, move your right hand forward (bum) and left knee following (BUM), then left hand (bum) and right knee following (BUM). Let your head lead your body so your back remains flat and stretched. Allow your hands and knees to stay close to the floor. Do not lift them too high as you are moving them forward.*

3. *Repeat any lines in iambic pentameter as you crawl, combining the rhythm of the iambics—bum BUM, bum BUM—with the landing of your hands and knees. Notice the feelings in your heart.*

4. *Now stand and recite the text, keeping in mind the organic movement of the crawling that you just explored. Feel how*

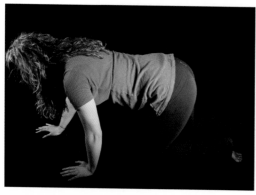

Crawling with the right hand leading.

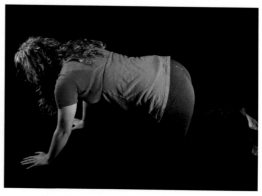

Crawling with the left hand leading.

having experienced the rhythm of your words physically in your body enlivens them when you speak them as text.

Moving horizontally is moving into activity on the earth. Moving vertically adds an element of spirituality, energy toward heaven. Traditional cultures teach the benefits of having a spine that is upright, to connect to earth from the base of the spine and to connect to heaven from the top of the head. Give your directions and do not diminish yourself by pulling muscles in and making yourself smaller as you go into activity.

After learning that crawling could help her have more feeling in her body, one student said to me, "Understanding crawling really helped me out. When you told me that iambic pentameter is like the human heartbeat, things fell into place. Shakespeare is nothing if not the human heart, and the iambic pentameter ties it all together. My whole body feels my heartbeat. It's not centralized. It's not cut off, and it is not a solo function. My heartbeat informs my breath, informs my thought, and informs my whole body to live in the text."

Crawling exercises can be used to prepare for any monologue. Before you speak, it is beneficial to be on your hands and knees and experience the lengthening and widening of your back in this position. Your movement can take on a sinuous or animal-like quality. Even though you would not do the crawling exercise on stage in performance, the exercise gives you information—information about how you are breathing, what your body is doing, and how you are connecting to what you are saying. Try the Counting Exercise to Explore Breath and Sound as you crawl.

Crawling also activates the cross-pattern reflex, which affects the development and growth of the nerve endings in the brain. This next variation connects the movement of your eyes and head to your torso. This is helpful for actors to train themselves to stay present in the room.

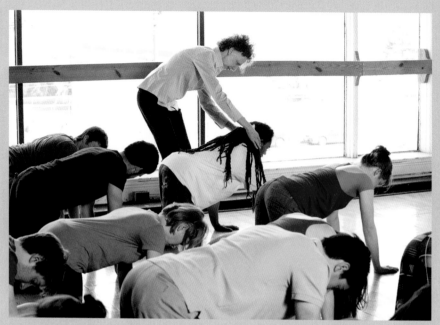
Help with crawling in a group.

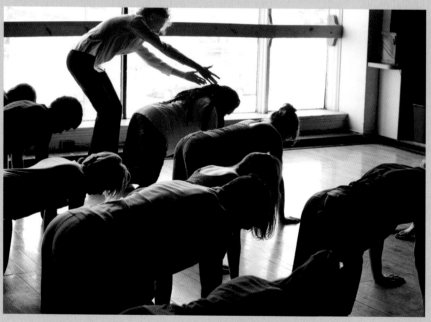
Group crawling.

Exercise to Explore Alexander Technique, Shakespeare, and Crawling, Engaging Your Eyes

We have looked at the involvement of your eyes starting from the top of your head and working our way down your body. In the Exercise to Explore Emotion and Breath, breathing in through the top of your nose, we explored the connection between the eyes, breath, and emotion. In the Exercise to Explore Whispered "Ah," we saw that your eyes are alive and sparkle as you exhale and vocalize. This exercise helps you coordinate your eye movement to the rest of your torso.

Preparation: *Perform any monologue.*

1. *Start on your hands and knees, palms under your shoulders and knees under your hips.*
2. *Turn your head and look at your right hand. Let your right hand and left knee move forward. Turn your head back to center.*
3. *Repeat the same process on other side, looking left, and then your left hand and right knee move forward. Look back to center and continue.*
4. *Try the process backward by looking to the side and stepping backward. Experiment with different combinations of moving and looking in different directions. Feel the creature-like quality of your body.*
5. *Return to your monologue and notice that your eyes now may feel more involved and activated in your monologue. Perhaps you are more receptive or more focused, or more connected to your body movements.*

After crawling, a student experienced the results of these exercises this way: "In doing Eleanor from *Henry VI Part II*, I found I didn't know what I was doing to my Gloucester or what I really wanted. As I gave my basic directions and allowed my whole body to become fully engaged, the monologue changed completely for me. My purpose became clear, my vision focused; my actions were more specific, and my whole self was involved." After she did the crawling exercise, she immediately stood up and spoke her text as her body continued to feel the sinuous motion inside.

Amount of Effort Needed to Convey a Character

It is not unusual for an actor to deliver a monologue using excess tension. We saw this in the Exercise to Explore Endgaining on Stage. Common examples of too much effort resulting in tension are scrunching your facial muscles in anger, lifting your shoulders in fear, or locking your knees in frustration. These habits have existed for generations.

I taught my work to Sydney Lemmon, actor Jack Lemmon's granddaughter, as a student in her junior year of acting training at Boston University. As she was dealing with her own issues of doing too much to convey a character (she was playing Juliet), she remembered a famous story of her grandfather. Jack Lemmon worked in the theater before he went into films. While working on a film, his director kept telling him "do less, do less" and finally in complete frustration he snapped and said, "If you make me do any less, I won't be doing anything at all." To which the director replied, "Exactly."[2] Having come from the theater, Jack was used to playing to big houses. Now working in front of the camera, there was much less effort needed to convey his story.

This anecdote also touches on Alexander's idea of "faulty sensory perception." What you think you are doing and what you are actually doing may be two different things. In Jack Lemmon's case, it may have felt like he was not doing anything, but in truth he was doing enough without adding any excess tension.

To explore this dilemma of faulty sensory perception in regard to how much effort you need, use these four steps as a general guideline:

1. Inhibit your immediate response as to what you think you need to do.
2. Give basic directions so that you use only as much tension as you need to convey the character.
3. Pull your head back as little as possible.
4. As the situation gets more intense, as it often does, you want to be able to have more intensity without having more tension in your body. Continue to stop and say no to your habit, go deeper inside, and then proceed from there. Be more aware of your sensations. There is a quality of suspended stillness in intensity.

To sort out the question of how much effort to use, it may be helpful to understand the nature of muscle fibers. There are two types of muscle fibers: the red, or slow-twitch fibers, are used for sustained activity. They work steadily over a long period of time and do not fatigue. They tend to be muscles that are closer to the bones. The white fast-twitch fibers are used for quick intense activity. They work hard and fast and then get tired. They tend to be more surface muscles. If you had more red slow-twitch fibers, you would be a good long distance runner. If you had more white fast-twitch fibers, you would be a good sprinter.

Many people today only use white fibers to move through life, doing strong movements and then collapsing. As a result, the red-fiber system has atrophied because of lack of use, which then makes standing or sitting for long periods of time seem like a difficult task; for some, it is impossible. The long-term overuse of the white-fiber muscles taxes the musculoskeletal, nervous, and circulatory systems. It might be a good idea at this point to reread chapter 5, "Suspension and Support," as it explains how standing off your support or standing without your suspension causes excess muscle tension.

Exercise to Explore Amount of Effort

Preparation: *Choose a piece of text or script with a character who has high stakes, a life-or-death situation. Go through the piece.*

1. *Stand as yourself and give your basic directions for suspension and support. This is a neutral position, which engages more red sustaining fibers. Your muscles in your back and legs are engaged but not working hard. There is no downward pull, which can be a strong interference when the red fibers are working properly.*

2. *Begin to think about your character and his or her situation, and let the white-fiber activity come in only as much as you need in the moment to convey what is going on. At this point, with certain emotions coming up, you might be tempted to overtense to express deep feelings. Instead, allow just enough muscular activity to convey the situation. If you are playing angry, you may tense your shoulders. But how much do you need to tense them? Saying "no" to habitual patterns allows something else to emerge.*

3. *Use your whole body, mind, and self to tell the story as you feel sensations inside. Feel what is going on inside, and speak from there. Let that have a voice. Let it vibrate, breathe, and emerge. Speak as if you are saying it for the first time. Say "no" to the habit. Be surprised. Go into the unknown. Too much white-fiber activity produces tension that will squeeze out creative impulses. Endgaining usually involves too much white-fiber activity.*

4. *As you run through the monologue or scene again, do not show what you are doing, but inhabit. Don't act an idea of what you think something is, just be it. Make sure your breath*

matches the situation. Know to whom you are talking and why. Let the intensity of the scene build without necessarily getting more tense. Remember the "Can I do less" portion of the Exercise to Explore Inhibition. Practice the Exercise to Explore Whispered "Ah" to connect to the amount of breath you need.

5. *As you do the monologue, notice the difference between dramatic tension and personal tension. Both can be using excess white fibers. Try the Exercise to Explore Inhibition: The Three Choices to see if you can make another choice. As an artist, you have a choice.*

Sometimes you are asked to play a character that is very tense or has compromised use, or has physical deformities. How do you play that day after day or night after night and not injure yourself? One student in every class will ask, "How do I play a character that has 'bad' use, such as Richard III?" You can use the Exercise to Explore Amount of Effort to explore moving with less effort to inform your choices. You want to try to get the physicality of the character first, without interfering with the creative process. Then keep the shape of the body, whatever that may be. Whatever shape you find yourself in, you can always give basic directions, and find the space within that shape and move from there.

The eloquent actress Mary Steenburgen has this to say: "Actors are constantly under some kind of stress—just the mere act, as Alexander found, of stepping out onto a stage is terrifying to some degree, for some of us more than for others. The question in terms of acting and the Alexander Technique for me was to be able to have some control over the tension. When you are playing a character that is pulled down, there is a way of being pulled down that is not necessarily in a slump. You can free your neck, allow your head to move forward and up and your whole body to follow, and still give the illusion of your character's physical tension or collapse.

It just requires experimenting and playing with it. An actor can learn to be hunched over without putting stress on his or her vocal mechanism. This is a very useful thing for a performer to know."[3]

Another student said, "Giving directions was hugely important for me in working on the play *Yerma*. I played Dolores, an old crone sorceress, and worked with a stooped physicality. Exploring the amount of effort helped me discover the character through my body, instead of trying to put a physicality on over myself. It also helped me live in that physicality without pain."

It is so tempting to do more than necessary when delivering a monologue or scene. It's common to do things like throw yourself off balance, overly tense muscles, or strain your voice. Instead, try saying "no" to these habits. Allow your surface white fibers to stop firing, and your deeper red fibers to engage. In other words, don't try to use more effort than is necessary to do the piece, but remember the Actor's Secret. Inhibit, direct, and see what is around you. Respond to that with the appropriate amount of effort.

CHAPTER 14

Scenes

The rehearsal process is a wonderful opportunity to explore possibilities of creative artistic expression with other actors. The principles of this book can enhance and enliven this process. In the rehearsal space, it's important for the cast and director to try to create an environment that allows the actors to be open and vulnerable, to be moved by the story. This allows the actors to experiment and to discover the value of inhibition, tracking, and proper breathing while in action.

As you do scene work, be sure that you are aware of yourself, and your character's needs, and at the same time listen to your scene partner's voice and body. An important part of this equation is the awareness of the physicality between you and your scene partners. The physicality includes your sensations, feelings, structure, and chemistry. How you use yourself to receive support from the ground and produce sound affects your scene partner.

When you have an ensemble made up of many people, it is important to understand the relationship of sound and voice among you. Explore the questions, "How does my voice affect you?" "Do you actually feel my voice or do you just hear it?" "What happens in your body as you feel my voice or just hear it?"

It is also important to be aware of support. Ask yourself, "When I let the ground support me, how does that affect you, my scene partner?" "If I let the ground support me while I speak, do I feel more powerful in my back?" "Can you feel what I'm saying in a more powerful way?" "Can you feel more sound vibrations?"

Exploring how you produce sound using your voice, and how you are aware of support as an ensemble, opens many possibilities.

It allows you to have your ground and your back, and there is less temptation to fall into habitual responses. If everybody in the ensemble is aware of their own support and their own back, everyone is connected with themselves, which leads to an overall coherence and connection, which produces cooperation to tell the story.

The first exercise in this chapter highlights the relationship of your feet to the ground. There are reflexes at the bottom of your feet between the long foot bones. Before the days of paved streets, when humans walked in the wild, it was absolutely necessary to engage these reflexes when walking on ground that was uneven. **As you walk on uneven ground, the reflexes in your feet tell the rest of your body how to balance and how to adjust to the uneven surface, or even to quicksand.** In most modern people these reflexes are atrophied, an unused resource. Thus there is limited contact and support from the ground. This exercise can help you improve your contact with the ground.

Exercise to Explore "Heels Down"

This exercise is done with a partner.

Preparation: *Sit for a moment in a chair by yourself with your feet touching the ground. Practice tracking the sensations in the bottoms of your feet. What do you feel? Can you feel that some parts of your foot rest on the ground and other parts pull away from the floor?*

Then explore what might change the contact your foot has with the ground. Try some other thoughts, like "I left my credit card at the restaurant." What happens to your feet? "This is the most beautiful sunset that I have ever seen." What happens to your feet? Are they tight? Lying flat? Lifting up?

Now choose a scene partner and a scene to work on.

1. *With both partners standing, exchange a few lines of text in a habitual way.*

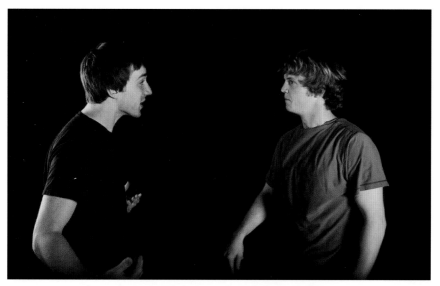

Exchange a few lines of text with a partner.

2. *Each person gives their own basic directions, and afterwards tries saying the same lines of text.*

3. *Explore steps 1 and 2 again, and notice if you are in contact with the ground with your feet. Notice the quality of contact.*

4. *Sit on the floor with the soles of your feet touching the soles of your partner's feet. Feel the sensation of what it feels like in your feet to touch your partner's feet.*

5. *Open and close your feet with your heels and toes together, then like windshield wipers, moving together back and forth. Try it about five times.*

6. *Gently push your feet back and forth, so your knees bend a little, keeping your soles together and heels on the floor. Try pushing against your partner's feet a little more, so your knees bend a lot.*

7. *Push more so you bend your knees and your feet come up off the floor. You both move your legs in the air while keeping the soles of your feet together. Explore your range.*

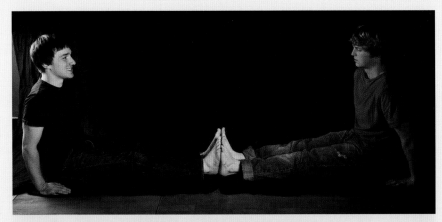

Put the soles of your feet together.

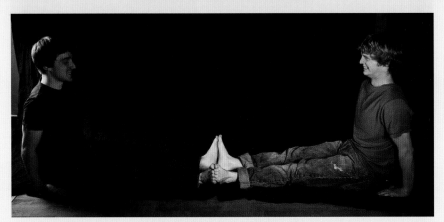

Open and close your feet.

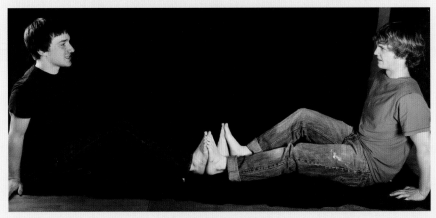

Gently push your feet.

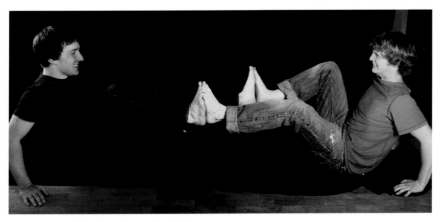

Explore your range.

8. *Return to step 4, having your feet together on the ground.*
9. *Separate from your partner's feet and put your feet on the floor. As you stand, can you now allow the ground to support you and feel the support coming up through your legs, spine, and head as we did in the Exercise to Explore Support?*
10. *Feel your feet in contact with the ground. Remember the mutual attraction between gravity and the earth. Notice how your feet feel. They may feel things like solid, freed, connected, or dropping into the ground.*
11. *Go back to the scene from the beginning of the exercise, and with your partner, say the lines of text. Notice the difference in sound and support after exploring the connection between your feet and the ground. Repeat the questions to your partner from the introduction to the chapter: "How does my voice affect you?" "Do you*

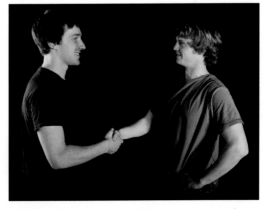

Return to the scene, noticing your connection to the ground.

actually feel my voice or do you just hear it?" "What happens in your body as you feel my voice or just hear it?"

You may notice that now you can connect to your partner through the floor. The same floor supports you. You may feel your feet sinking into the ground. This gives you tremendous support, which makes you unshakeable. When you are so rooted in yourself and to the ground, you can really communicate with others. Notice the quality of your voice now.

After exploring this exercise, students have said things like, "I learned that I did not need to fidget." "I have less head-bobbing." "I have a more focused voice." and "I am more involved in the story."

The second exercise to explore scene work highlights the importance of your back. Your back includes your whole torso and your spine or backbone. You have heard the expression "spineless" or

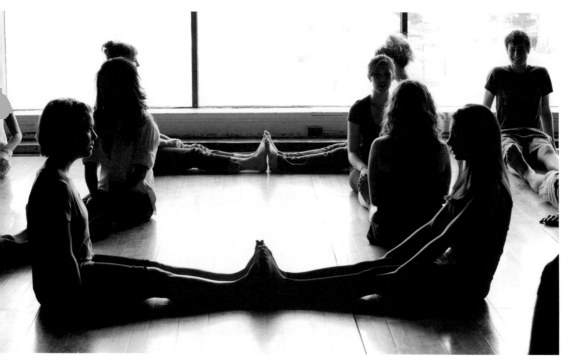

Group class exploring Heels Down.

"the backbone of society." These expressions imply that strength of character is a reflection of the strength of your back. Learn to engage your back. As you become aware of the presence of your back, you will feel more connected to yourself and to your inherent strength and power. This is a valuable tool both on stage and off.

Exercise to Explore Staying in Your Back

This exercise is done with a partner.

Preparation: *As you sit by yourself, practice tracking the sensations in your back. What parts of your back feel held or tight? What parts feel free?*

Then explore thoughts that might change your back: "Sit up straight." What happens in your back? "I have not eaten and feel weak." What happens in your back?

Now choose a partner close to your height, and exchange a few lines from a scene.

1. *Sit on a cushion on the floor or on a chair with your back against your partner's back.*

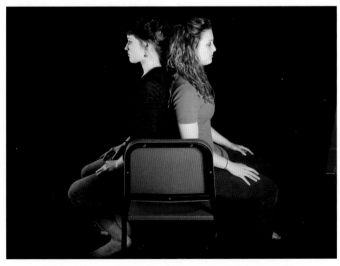

Sit with your back touching your partner's back.

~ 205 ~

2. *Feel the support of your partner's back against yours. Does that help you feel the backward dimension that we explored in the Exercise to Explore Three-Dimensional Breathing?*

3. *Don't push too hard, but be sure to have some contact with each other. Lean into the other person. Feel your back.*

4. *Lock elbows and rock forward and backward with your backs touching.*

5. *Move side to side with your backs touching.*

6. *Do a whispered "ah" together and feel the aim up of your back. Try to have the feeling of falling up. Feel your own back and your partner's back.*

7. *Now try a vocalized "ah." Then try vocalizing each vowel sound: "ah," "eh," "ee," "oh," "oo." Feel the vibration in your back, and in your partner's back.*

8. *Aim your head up.*

9. *Allow your belly to drop into your back as you exhale, vocalizing some of the vowels again.*

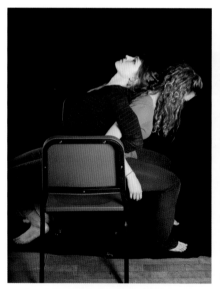 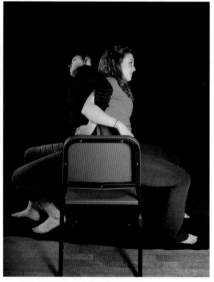

| Rock forward and back with your backs touching. | Move side to side with your backs touching. |

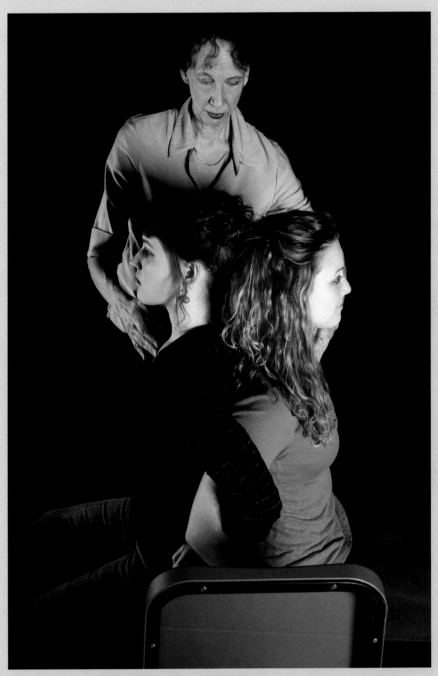

Aim up along your spine as you exhale so that your spine is poised,
alert, and directed.

10. *Now stand, and notice how your back feels.*

11. *Try the scene again with your partner and notice your back and your partner's back, and your resonant sound and support. Repeat the questions from the introduction to the chapter: "When I let the ground support me, how does that affect you, my scene partner?" "If I let the ground support me while I speak, do I feel more powerful in my back?" "Can you feel what I am saying in a more powerful way?" "Can you feel more sound vibrations?"*

Bringing attention and feeling to your back this way can allow you to feel your own power and bigness. This fills you and the room with your presence.

After doing this exercise, one student said, "I found my back and I felt like I remembered who I was. I felt like I owned myself again. I was okay with being alone and not afraid of it. I felt tall, big, beautiful, and powerful. Later that day I worked on a scene playing Joan of Arc, and was able to take up the whole room without worrying about being too big, both physically and vocally."

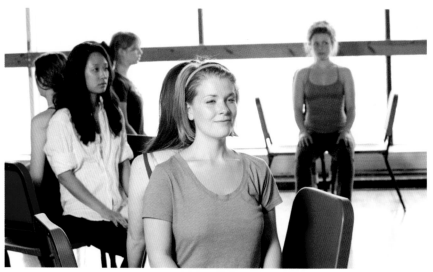

Group exploring Staying in Your Back.

When you combine the Exercise to Explore "Heels Down" and the Exercise to Explore Staying in Your Back while giving directions, and add a playful quality to it, you can expand your choices and free up your creativity and imagination. It is important to play in a light-hearted way and have fun sometimes to free your energy.

Exercise to Explore "Heels Down, Stay Back, Aim Up"

This exercise is done with a group.

Preparation: *This exercise can be done with two or more people. If you're in rehearsal for a play, try the scene with the ensemble.*

1. *Do the Exercise to Explore "Heels Down" with a partner.*
2. *Now try the Exercise to Explore Staying in Your Back with a partner.*
3. *Now everyone makes a circle, and give your basic directions.*
4. *Allow your heels to drop, so that you are not leaning forward ("heels down"). Stay lengthened and widened in your back, so that you are not narrowing ("stay back"). Aim up, so that you are not dropping down ("aim up"). Repeat the phrase "heels down, stay back, aim up."*
5. *Walk around the room repeating the phrase.*
6. *Explore on your own "heels down, stay back, aim up" in various activities, real or imagined.*
7. *With the ensemble, take turns with each person calling out an activity, like skip. The person who called it out says, "As I skip: heels down, stay back, aim up." Then the group repeats the phrase as they do the activity.*

Other activities can be: "I am dancing with my partner: heels down, stay back and aim up." The group partners up and repeats the phrase as they dance. This helps you to be aware of your feet

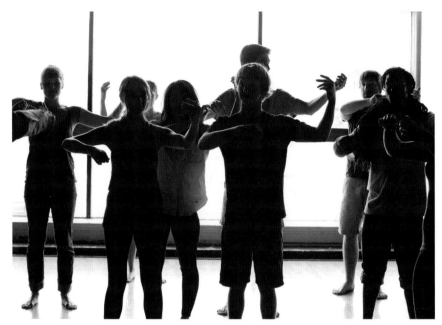

"Heels Down, Stay Back, Aim Up" as I play the violin.

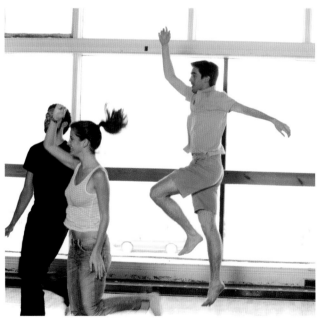

"Heels Down, Stay Back, Aim Up" as I skip.

on the ground, the presence of your back, and your aim up as you speak and do the activity.

Some other examples of activities to try are singing, playing an instrument, talking on the phone, or imaginary actions like eating a doughnut or playing kickball as you say, "heels down, stay back, aim up."

After you complete the exercise, try enacting a scene with a partner. Notice the changes in creativity and imagination as well as in support and sound.

Exercise to Explore Connection through Sensation

This exercise is done with a partner.

The acting profession brings you in touch with many different kinds of people. We all have preferences concerning who we feel connected to and who we would like to spend time with. **Sometimes you need to do a scene with someone you do not feel connected to, or with someone you don't feel comfortable with.** This exercise can help build a new bridge of connection. Do this exercise with someone you are working on a scene with. As you prepare for this exercise, you may want to remember the Exercise to Explore Boundaries to be aware of your personal space comforts.

Part 1:

Preparation: *To remind yourself of the maximum extension of your arms, reach your arms out to the sides, as you did in the Exercise to Explore Hands on the Back of the Chair.*

1. *Do a scene with your partner.*
2. *After the scene, take a moment to stand. Extend your arms all around you: in front, above, and behind you. This establishes what is called your **kinesphere**. It is the space within*

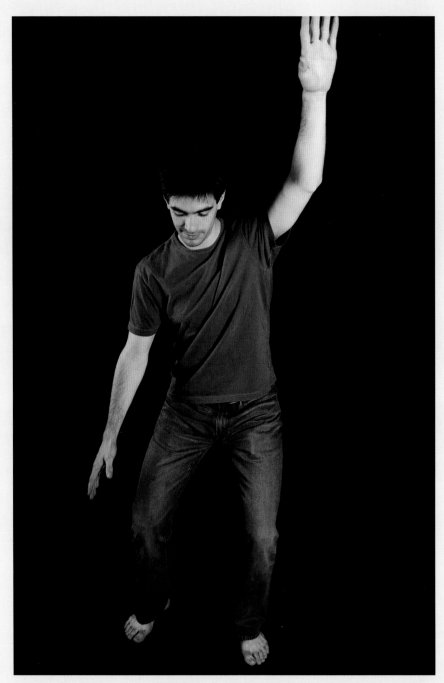

Establish your kinesphere.

your reach as you stand. Notice the sensations in your body as you reach in different directions.

3. *With your scene partner, decide who is A and who is B. Partner A: move in and out of Partner B's kinesphere without touching your partner.*

4. *Both partners: notice what it is like to have someone close to you, coming in and out of your personal space. What happens to your breath? Notice the sensations in your body. Notice how your senses become heightened. Notice how you know when someone is behind you. Remember what you noticed in the Exercise to Explore Boundaries.*

5. *Now try switching roles, Partner B stepping into Partner A's kinesphere. Notice that a sensory bond has been established between you and your partner.*

6. *Do the scene again, using the sensory information you may have learned from being in your partner's kinesphere. Your bodily and sensory awareness may be heightened. Colors may seem brighter and impulses more visceral and stronger.*

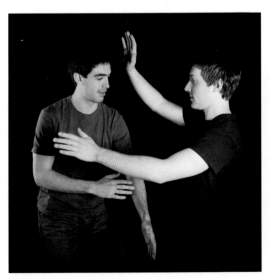

Explore moving in your partner's kinesphere.

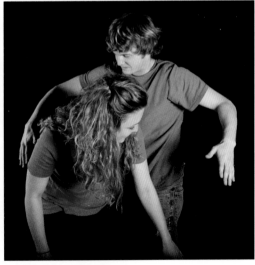

Explore moving in your partner's kinesphere as you track your sensations.

Part 2:

To deepen the connection, with the same partner, choose roles: Partner A is watching and Partner B is being watched.

1. *Sit across from your partner and observe your partner from a distance, in relationship to the walls and the surrounding environment. Notice the sensations in your body. What is your "gut" feeling as you notice your partner? What happens to your heartbeat?*

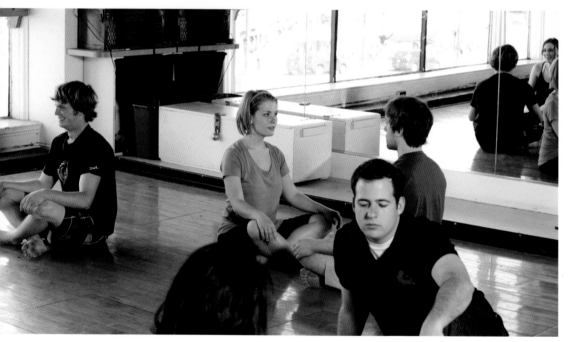
Observe your partner.

2. *Partner A: move around and see Partner B in different backgrounds. Observe five or six details about your partner, like her smile, her hair, the buttons on her shirt. What happens in your body? Track your sensations.*

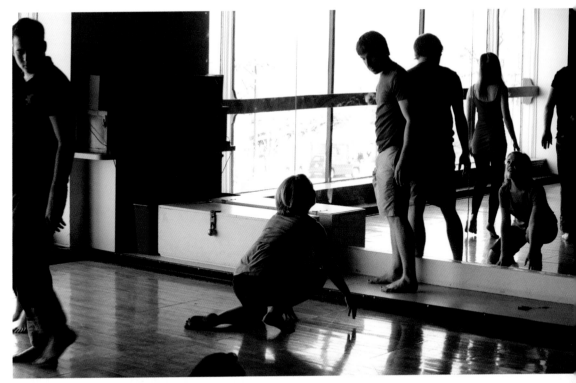

Observe your partner as he or she moves.

3. As Partner A moves around, the background behind Partner B changes. Notice these details as the environment changes.
4. Partner A: choose one detail that is distinct about your partner. Notice that detail in a changing environment as Partner B is moving around the room. What happens in your body?
5. Partner A: move apart from your partner so that you do not see her, but continue to think about her and especially keep the thoughts in mind and the sensations in your body of the one detail you chose.
6. Reunite with your partner and notice the heightened connection.
7. Switch roles.

8. Run through the scene taking into account what you learned from establishing this new connection through sensation.

Many students have said that they feel connected to their scene partner in a way that they never imagined after doing this exercise. A close bond is developed on a human sensory level. If it is not possible to do this exercise with your scene partners, then try the following exercise.

Working with a Diva or Someone You Perceive to Be Better Than You

With certain people, you might tend to make them out to be larger, or more powerful, than you. This in turn seemingly makes you smaller and less powerful. Of course, in the bigger picture, no one person is better than another, even if they happen to be famous. But it's easy to be overwhelmed by big personalities or strong egos.

This exercise involves imagination. The mind is a powerful entity. However, we often unwittingly end up using it in a negative cycle, working against ourselves. You can imagine something, and even if it is not true, your body will respond accordingly. If you imagine that you walk into an audition and choke on your lines in fear, your body will respond accordingly and tense up. But we can also use this response in a positive way to relieve distressing symptoms and promote a corrective experience. You can imagine a situation and respond in a new, more positive way. For example, if you imagine going into the audition and doing a fantastic job, your body will feel relaxed, confident, and upbeat.

Exercise to Explore Working with a Diva or Difficult Personality

Part 1: Distance Yourself from the Situation

Preparation: *When there is danger close by, it can be very disturbing to a person. If you can create some distance between yourself and the danger, some relief from the fear is possible. You can deal with the fear in smaller doses. Sit in a space that feels safe to you. Feel your ground, your breath, and your back. You can have your eyes open or closed.*

1. *Picture yourself walking onto the set or rehearsal room and seeing a person who makes you uncomfortable. Feel the jolt of fear that might make you want to hit him or her (fight), run from him or her (flight), or become catatonic (freeze). Get to know your own pattern.*

2. *Where is the tension in your body? What does it make your body do? Does it make your legs stiffen? Your shoulders lift? Your gut wrench?*

3. *"Be with" the somatic experience as you continue to imagine the difficult person. Come in touch with sensations that are just below the surface of your consciousness. You may feel muscular twitches, you may even hear screaming inside that wants to be voiced. Let your body follow these twitches with small, slow movements that arise from within. Feel the root of the impulse, and shift it a little bit. Let your voice produce a quieter version of the scream, perhaps "gr-r-r" or "a-a-ah" to unroot it.*

4. *Notice any small moments of relief and allow them to metabolize in your whole body. Recognize that your feet are on the ground and let the ground support you. Let that support radiate up through your whole body, and let your back fill with your own self-generated energy. Notice your breathing now. Is your breath flowing more fully? Are your ribs moving?*

5. *Now try pendulating back and forth between feeling the fear and then feeling the relief a few times before you move on.*

6. *As you imagine the diva now, can you see him or her as a bit smaller and see yourself a bit bigger and fuller?*

Repeat Part 1 of the exercise a few times until you feel even a tiny bit less intimidated by the strong personality.

Part 2: On the Set or In Rehearsal

After you have successfully worked with your diva partner from a distance, try this sequence when you next come into contact with him or her.

1. *Next time you walk onto the set or into the rehearsal room and see him or her, you may feel your familiar fear patterns arise from the exercise above. If those feelings do arise, stay with yourself and track your sensations.*

2. *When those sensations settle down a little, choose one detail that you like about the person. Maybe he or she has a funny smile, her hair curls nicely today, or he's wearing a shirt that's a nice shade of blue. These observations can be a resource that connects you to the present moment and helps you find a little more comfort within yourself.*

3. *Let your body feel and respond to the present moment with something comforting that you like—the resource. Let your body metabolize that comfortable feeling.*

4. *You may pendulate back and forth between feeling the fear and the comfort a few times before you are able to settle and feel the kind of support that no one can take away. Then you can land in a productive place to act from.*

This sequence takes only a few moments and can greatly reduce the stress that can interfere with your acting. As you go through the exercise, remember to feel the strength of your spine, and stay present with the full stature of yourself.

Because long hours of rehearsals or shooting can be tiring, you need to be able to use your energy wisely. Using your ground for support and your back for strength opens your energy channels. As you practice the scene-work exercises in this chapter, your acting will have more depth, and you will feel a more dynamic and appropriate physicality in your scenes. The body comes alive when it is honest. Let your body find the truth. Hear the truth of what is happening to you.

CHAPTER 15

Auditions

Auditioning is an opportunity to show yourself and your skills. Yet most actors are not able to make the most of this opportunity because they get frozen or seized with fear. **Just the word** *audition* **seems to make most actors nervous.** It brings up self-doubt and questions self-worth. Because of this, auditions tend to trigger major fear responses.

The following exercises will help you understand your own fear responses. The major fear responses are fight, flight, and freeze. These are part of the defensive reflex responses, which are a part of the evolution of adaptive social behavior. When there is danger, your impulse is either to fight the danger, run to escape the danger, or to freeze to be invisible to the danger, in order to try to defend yourself.

It is noteworthy to mention that research by Stephen W. Porges, a neuroscientist and director of the Brain-Body Center at the University of Illinois, has named what is called "the social engagement system." This system is part of his Polyvagal Theory, a theory that links the evolution of the vertebrate autonomic nervous system to the emergence and neurobiology of social behavior. This hierarchal system has three steps: the first is your ability to engage socially with people around you. Your facial muscles are very involved and expressive in this contact. When there is the possibility of danger, your facial muscles try to identify if there is actually danger present. The second step emerges if a person or situation is actually dangerous and you need to defend yourself. Your fight or flight response kicks in. If they fail to defend you and the situation is life-threatening, the body goes into shutdown mode, or freeze, which is the third stage. When the danger is over, your face responds, perhaps with a smile or a look of relief, and you are back in social engagement—back to step one, until the next danger comes along.

Each of us has our own combination of responses to a fearful situation. It is helpful to practice a fake audition to see what particular fear responses come up for you and what you can do about them. This can be done in a group or alone. Exploring fear responses in a group is more effective because it is usually the other people who "make" you nervous. Thus many students say, "When I'm at home and say my lines with no one else around, the script sounds fine and I am not nervous." So what causes the nervousness when you get into the audition setting?

Explanation of Reflex Responses

There are two major attitudinal reflex responses in humans: the startle reflex and the righting reflex. The startle reflex occurs when you are surprised. A startle occurs with anything from a door slamming to a tiger jumping out at you. A startle also occurs when you think someone is judging you or criticizing you. When you are frightened or nervous, there is a particular bodily response that includes pulling the head back and down, pulling the shoulders up, and locking the knees. This is your body preparing to deal with the fearful situation. Because you may be in danger, the startle reflex leads to defensive orienting responses such as fight, flight, or freeze. Frank Pierce Jones, a well-known Alexander teacher who did research on the scientific validity of the Alexander Technique, wrote about the startle reflex. "The change, which is not instantaneous, begins in the head and neck, passing down the trunk and legs to be completed in about half a second."[1]

The second major reflex response is the righting reflex. The righting reflex occurs when the body returns to a state of peaceful equilibrium or equipoise. All the muscles are extended equally, each

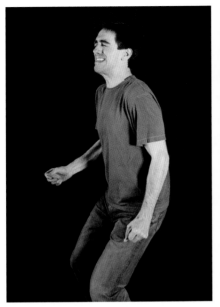

The startle reflex.

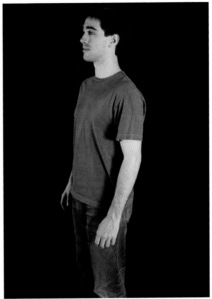

The righting reflex.

working just a bit, nothing working too much or too little. When the righting reflex is engaged, you feel balanced and peaceful.

We can see both of these responses in the animal kingdom by observing a cat. The cat can be lazing around the window on a sunny day enjoying the warmth (righting reflex). Then it sees a mouse and its body stiffens as it prepares for fight or flight (startle reflex). The mouse runs away, and the cat returns to lazing by the window (righting reflex). Modern life is full of startle, starting with the alarm clock that wakes you up. Even the word *alarm* tells you what kind of reflex it might provoke.

The first component of the startle reflex, when examined with multistrobe photography, is the head moving back and down. This reflex works in two directions: when you go into startle, your head moves back and down; and when your head moves back and down, that can also cause you to go into startle. Many people often put themselves into startle by pulling their head back and down, and feel the fear and anxiety that accompanies the reflex, even though there is nothing directly to fear in that moment.

The startle reflex is not a bad thing. It is a very important reflex for survival. Fear used well is a good thing. We are not trying to get rid of a startle pattern, but rather trying to reevaluate what we see as real danger. The audition room is not the modern version of the tiger . . . although the actor sometimes feels that it is.

Righting Reflex

The righting reflex is the ability to assume an optimal position when there has been a departure from it. Life circumstances often throw the body off balance. In the animal kingdom, the righting reflex is a cat's innate ability to orient itself as it falls in order to land on its feet. We can use a similar analogy in humans. You are often thrown emotionally and need to land quickly on your feet. Metaphorically, this is a common occurrence in auditions.

In humans the reflex is constantly adjusting muscles and bones to maintain uprightness and equilibrium. When you stand and move your hip to one side, you will see that your rib cage automatically moves to the opposite side to balance you, and your neck tilts in the same direction as your hip. This automatic reflex—the resulting tilt in posture—is trying to maintain your head over your cervical spine (your neck), your eyes level to the horizon, and your weight over your feet for your support, so that you don't fall over.

When you go to an audition, you want to feel comfortable with yourself and the space around you. When you are thrown off balance and feel anxious, it's hard to feel comfortable. One way to increase your comfort and decrease your anxiety is to find a way to feel safe. **Looking around the room to orient yourself to your surroundings is one way to feel safe.** As you feel safe, your body is able to right itself. This means that you can feel a sense of equipoise, and remember that all your muscles are working equally to balance you.

Exercise to Explore Righting Reflex to Orient Yourself

This exercise can help you get better at orienting yourself in new places and situations.

Preparation: *Sit in a comfortable chair. Let your feet be on the ground and let your back touch the back of the chair.*

1. *As you sit, notice your breathing.*
2. *Allow your neck to be free.*
3. *Turn your head slowly to the right.*
4. *As you are turning, allow your eyes to take in the environment. Do not squint or try to see. Take your time.*
5. *Return your head to center.*
6. *Do the same as you turn your head to the left. It is important that you allow your eyes to go where they want. You want to be sensing more than thinking.*
7. *Feel what happens in your body as you realize that there is no danger.*
8. *Return your head to center. Notice your breathing now.*

You can use this exercise to minimize anxiety and feel safe. You can do it before your audition, or as you are waiting to perform. **This process allows you to feel ease within yourself, which is different from being relaxed or collapsed.**

Startle Reflex

Earlier in this book, we looked at overwhelming experiences, and the examples of the rabbit and the woman biking to work. We saw that **the defensive reflex responses need to be completed so that the nervous system and body are not compromised in their function.** These defensive responses are designed to operate for a short period of time. They are time-limited—they defend you and they finish, designed to pass once the threat is over. But when they are not completed, they continue to fire inaccurate messages: they tell you there is danger when there isn't any. This results in dysregulation in the autonomic nervous system. That is why we see symptoms in the body related to breathing, muscle holding, and more. When the nervous system is compromised, a symptom of that is anxiety. Here are three stories displaying what can happen when the three major defensive fear responses—fight, flight, and freeze—have not been completed. These stories can be used to understand your own responses, or the responses of your character.

Fight

One young actor I worked with was always arguing and disagreeing with people in his daily life. He had an edge that was unpleasant to be around, always looking for a fight. He happened to get cast as a pleasant person, so he came to me for coaching.

As he sat, I asked him to pay attention to his body. He said that he could feel that his upper body was tight, and he could not feel his legs. As I asked him to sense his legs, he said he felt something pulling his legs up off the ground. He felt anxious, with his arms tight, like he would feel before a fight. He breathed out after he said that. He said, "I needed to clench my feet because the world was cramming down on me; I had to fight back. My shoulders and arms were always ready for a fight. I had to fight to stay alive." His home life had been difficult as a child and he felt like he had to work and fight for his survival. After he was able to express his realizations, his feet became warm as the energy returned, and he felt his support from the ground for the first time. He stood and walked around the room, saying his feet felt like wings opening. He gave his directions, and then he felt his head release up, his arms release out, and his feet suction to the ground. He was now very stable, and not at all looking for a fight. His face lit up as his social engagement system kicked in. He was excited to go to rehearsal that night. As we studied in chapter 9, "Voice," regarding the omohyoid muscle, any shoulder tension will hinder your voice.

When you explore, in yourself or in a character, the qualities of an incomplete fight response, you will often find tight neck and shoulders. The actor in the above story walked around most of his life with his arms and shoulders tight, just waiting to punch somebody. This exercise is not about punching pillows to release tension, but instead, feeling the impulses and small movements, so that you can free them from holding. Punching pillows expresses the anger; feeling the impulse or sensation allows you to experience or be with the anger.

Flight

A student I worked with who was in her mid-twenties was having problems with her legs. They were often very tight and cramping, and it was hard for her to stand for long periods of time on stage. As it turned out, she revealed to me that she had been molested at age ten, and had tried to run away but could not. Fifteen years later, her legs were still trying to discharge the energy of running away. After we worked, exploring her boundaries, being with the leg tension, and moving it through, her legs stopped cramping and her stage work improved. She was able to do the Exercise to Explore Monkey to get more fluidity in her legs and connect to the ground.

A person or a character with an incomplete flight response will often have tight legs. At some point the legs wanted to run to help escape a dangerous situation. This can turn into restless leg syndrome (when the legs want to run or move constantly, so they shake or bounce), or the tightness can interfere with your acting.

Freeze

Sally was playing the role of a queen. As a queen, she needed to be bold and speak her mind. But every time she had to speak boldly, she froze. She felt a knot in her solar plexus that would not move. It was a familiar pattern. She came for a lesson and I asked her to describe the knot. As she was describing it, she had an image of her father's stern face and she felt helpless, and unable to speak up. As she kept her attention on the knot, she said the strands began to unwind. Her body had unconsciously been holding on to this freezing pattern. She said, "I feel like I am growing on the inside. I feel all of me. I am now able to express anger, sadness, and pain. I am not afraid to speak."

The person or character with an incomplete freeze response will often hold back physically and emotionally. They often have frozen feelings that include contractions or "knots" in muscles or internal organs. Also, an unfulfilled freeze response can result in a feeling of immobility in the whole body, resulting in a limited capacity to move. The Exercise to Explore a Stuck Place can be very helpful with this pattern.

These three stories give us a vivid picture of what can happen when defensive responses are not completed. Understanding these patterns is an invaluable tool for an actor. Levine wrote, "If a posture is rigid from bracing or is collapsed, we can assume it was a preparation for some particular action, an action that was thwarted and that the muscles are still programmed to complete."[2] The following exercise gives you an opportunity to discover your version of the startle pattern and your common defensive patterns.

Exercise to Explore the Startle Reflex and Performance Anxiety

This exercise is done with a group.

Part 1:

Preparation: *Sit in a circle.*

1. *Go around the circle naming your typical fear responses. "When I am nervous or getting ready to go on stage, I have ____ (sweaty palms, a racing heart, leg cramps, butterflies in my stomach, dry mouth, I talk a lot)." As you hear the responses, you see that most people have some kind of fear patterns that disempower them. You may be able to notice that some of your patterns connect to what you observed in the Exercise to Explore Your Identifications.*

2. *Set up a space of an audition room with a door to walk in and a row of chairs for the auditioners. One actor stands*

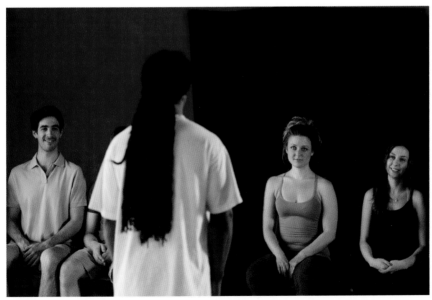

Standing in front of the audition panel.

outside the door and the others sit in the chairs as the audition panel.

3. *The actor who is outside the door can now walk into the room and face the panel and say, "My name is ____ (Tim). I will sing ____ ('The Rose')." The actor will not be singing, but the thought will often elicit a fear response.*

4. *Take turns; each person has a chance to come into the room. Announce your name and what you are going to perform. After you speak, sit down and write three fear responses that happened for you when you were in front of the audition panel, or even on entering the room. Some common physical fear responses that might have come up are heart racing, sweating, twitching, neck tightening, nausea, tight gut, butterflies in your stomach, feeling like you can't breathe, shoulders tensing up, mouth getting dry, tongue feeling stuck in throat, feeling like you can't think.*

Part 2:

Preparation: *Prepare for lying-down work on the floor with a book under your head, knees bent, and feet flat.*

1. *Give basic directions: Allow your neck to be free, allow your head to free forward and up, allow your back to lengthen and widen, and allow the ground to support you.*

2. *Notice that you are not in the audition room anymore. You are alone now with nobody watching you or evaluating you. What happens in your body?*

3. *Think about entering the audition room—notice what happens. Specifically notice any tension in your neck.* **The neck houses three important passageways: the trachea for air, the esophagus for food, and the spine, which houses the nervous system.**

4. *Starting with the front of your neck, allow your trachea to free. In the middle of your neck, allow the esophagus to be free. In the back of your neck, allow your spine to be free. It is very important not to constrict these functions.*

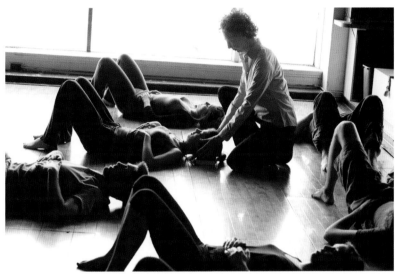

Lying down with basic directions.

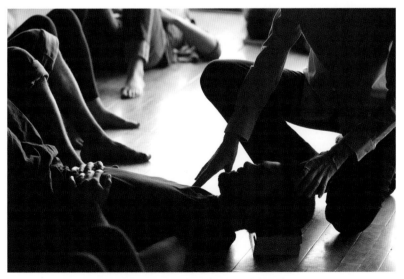

Allowing your neck to be free, lying down.

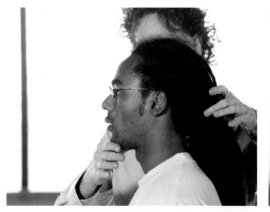

Allowing the neck to be free, standing.

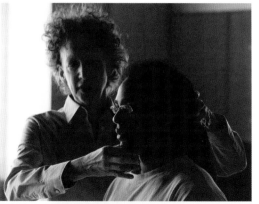

Allow the head to release forward and up.

5. *One of the major patterns we see in the fear response is interference with the flow of breath.* Interference often results in needing to lift your shoulders to take an accessory breath. As you are lying on the floor, put one hand on your belly and one hand on your ribs, and allow them to move as you breathe. Do not lift your shoulders. Do the silent "la la la" to get a maximum exhale so that you then get a reflex inhale.

6. Now think about walking into the audition room as you let your neck be free, let the floor support you, and allow your breath to flow in and out.

7. Make your way to standing and return to the set-up audition room.

8. Each person enters the room again. This time, before you walk into the room, orient, stay in your back, breathe, and find your support. Walk to the center of the panel and repeat the phrase, "My name is ____ (Tim). I will sing ____ ('The Rose')."

9. If fear arises, have the thought, "I'm nervous, but I can still breathe and expand." Remember your field of energy bubble.

As you walk into the audition room, if you pull your head back, it is like putting yourself in startle reflex and putting on the brakes. Instead, allow your head to free forward and up, and then you can accelerate with full life-force energy. Open to the fear and embrace it. When you audition this way, you are present and free from excess fear responses. You have a healthy excitement that is directed into your performance. The audition panel sees you as alive and vibrant without your characteristic fear responses crippling you.

The audition process is such an important part of an actor's life and career. Take the time to explore the above sequence. If you're not in a group, try it anyway, imagining the group there.

Here are three stories about auditioning that demonstrate how saying "no" to the habitual, using the silent "la la la," and "being with" can help you with your audition process.

"When I was in high school, I had crippling stage fright that I would always get before auditions. In many auditions I would completely lose the words and make an utter fool of myself. This work helped me to say 'no' to that and explore other options. During auditions, I knew well in advance that I would get nervous, and that would cause me to severely mess up. In the audition, the second I noticed my heart quickening, I went to my Actor's Secret 'tool bag,' and my attention went straight to the ground. I allowed myself to breathe regularly and I simply focused on the moment—not thinking of the past or future, and allowed myself to just be. My nerves were totally calmed and the audition went well."

"When I audition, finding my breath and using the silent "la la la" has become increasingly beneficial for me in speaking, singing, and dancing. When I do the breath work, I feel grounded, strong, open, and vulnerable. I went on an open-call audition in New York and made it to the final round. I used my basic directions and the breath work. I felt comfortable about my performance and a strange sense of relaxation when I finished. I did my best. There was nothing more I could have done. When I was called back again, instead of getting nervous, I became more relaxed. **I do not know how or why, but the breathing restored my faith in myself.**"

One student came to see me the day after a big audition and told me she had post-audition anxiety. She said that she felt pain in her back. I asked her to describe the pain to me. She said she felt twitches and some trembling. I asked her to "be with" the twitches. They stopped, and her back began to feel wide. Then her breath expanded. She said, "The anxiety is still there but it's not overtaking me. I have chronic anxiety and I have always tried to shove it away. But ironically, when I stayed with it, it subsided. Now when I think about the audition, I want to laugh. There will be another one."

I have spent most of the audition chapter explaining what anxiety looks and feels like. In my experience, it is important for you to understand the cause of your anxiety and take the steps necessary to work with it. That will enable you to say "no" to your habitual use and behavior and make choices based on the circumstances in the present moment. Then your skill and talent as an actor is there to help you perform your audition to the best of your ability.

In a master class, the well-known actor Kevin Spacey spoke about auditions. "Don't let your own judges lead you to panic. Don't try to be what you think they want. Instead, recognize **that they have a problem:** they need an actor. They want someone to solve the problem. **You may be the solution.** Be yourself. That is enough."[3]

CHAPTER 16

Taking the Stage

As you make your way through to the process of performance, from the audition to the rehearsal room to the stage or set, each step reveals new circumstances and new stimuli. In a performance there is a large added stimulus. People are paying attention to you, watching every move you make, usually paying money to see you. How do you respond?

If your response is to shrink and become smaller, you block off parts of yourself, both muscularly and energetically. Then these parts cannot participate in the performance, either mentally or physically. If you can inhibit your habitual response to close down, and instead stay open to your expanded self, you may be pleasantly surprised by what you find or what finds you. Invite the process of being seen, even if it is scary. Remember your suspension, find your support, and see what is around you.

In daily life many tall or largely built people tend to try to make themselves look smaller, by hunching down, pulling in their energy, or sucking in the stomach. On stage, an actor with this habit of making himself small has a dilemma. If he follows his habit and becomes smaller, he needs to do a lot of big gestures to try to convey an idea. But instead, if he gives his directions, he allows himself to get bigger and own his full stature. From full stature there is no need for overdoing. A small gesture becomes very powerful.

As you open yourself to your full stature, you may feel some fear. To deal with the fear that may emerge when you stay open, use the tools we have discussed in previous chapters: breath, directions, improved use, "be with," and support. When you are supported by these tools, you will find that you have less need and desire to hold onto the fear that you thought you needed. You can then be more present for the performance.

In the performance space, you want to have an awareness of the whole room, including all four corners of the room. There are most likely two corners you see and two you do not see. Keeping an awareness of the entire room keeps your attention expanded, so that you may be less likely to pull in or make yourself smaller. As you sense the space, you know what is in it, including other actors and the audience, or the crew, as the case may be. Even without looking at the audience, you develop a relationship with them. There is some kind of flow of energy between an actor and the audience in this expanded field of attention.

In performance, there is a dynamic between the actor and the audience. The concept of dynamic opposition is important here. It is the idea that two objects or parts have some pull flowing between them. Every performer knows that feeling of something magnetic between himself or herself and the audience or camera. There are also oppositions within the body to explore. Exploring dynamic oppositions in the body can increase awareness of dynamic oppositions with the audience.

Oppositions in the Body

Many oppositions exist in the body. Within your body you can allow your head to free away from your spine, and you experience opposition between your head and your spine. Your arms and legs oppose your torso.

There are oppositions between your body and something outside, like your feet opposing the floor. There is also a powerful opposition between the bodies of two actors on stage. The idea of opposition creates an interaction between parts, which brings aliveness, support, and suspension. This idea helps a stage actor become large and fill the space without getting tense. Oppositions can give someone acting on the set a strong sense of presence to create a dynamic with the camera.

Exercise to Explore Oppositions

Part 1:

Preparation: *To feel oppositions within your body, sit in a chair in a comfortable space.*

1. *Notice what happens as you sit habitually. Perhaps you pull your head back, or shorten your back, or lift your feet off the floor.*

Try sitting in the chair with these oppositions:

2. *Let your feet oppose the ground. This means your feet are in contact with the ground, not pressing hard or pulling away. Once you receive that contact, you free away from it to oppose it.*
3. *Let your hips oppose the chair. This means that your sitting bones are in contact with the chair and you let the chair support you.* **When your sitting bones are in touch with the chair, there is no need to tighten your hip sockets or your legs.**

Part 2:

Start by standing. Then try moving to sit in the chair with these oppositions:

1. *Take your head forward (do not pull it back.) Feel your head forward in relationship to your back moving back.*
2. *Take your back backward (do not let your back collapse forward) in relationship to your head freeing forward.*
3. *Take your knees slightly forward (do not pull them back). Feel them forward in relationship to your heels freeing back.*

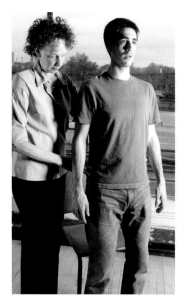 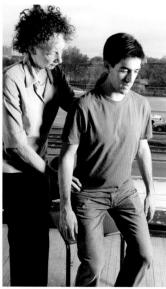 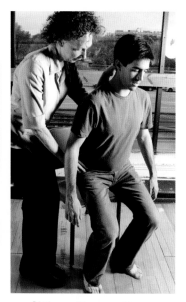

| Standing with oppositions. | Knees and nose ease forward. Back and heels ease back. | Sitting with oppositions. |

4. *Take your heels back. Feel them back in opposition to your knees. Do not go forward on your toes.*

5. *Now remove the chair and try bending, knees bending forward and lowering down as if you were going to pick something up off the floor. Find oppositions as you bend. Your knees and nose go forward; your back and heels go back. You will recognize that the oppositions are defining the muscular pulls in the Exercise to Explore Monkey.*

Part 3:

Preparation: *To get more feeling of the oppositional pulls, go to a door and open it, then take hold of both handles.*

1. *Lean your back away from the door. Feel your back opposing the door.*

2. *Bend and straighten your knees and keep your back opposing the door.*

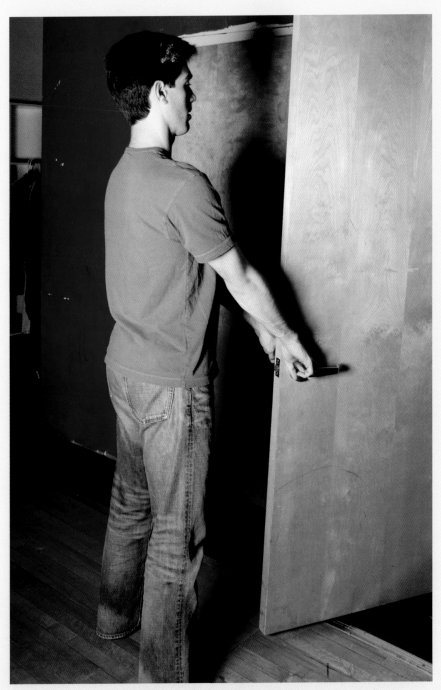

Lean your back away from the door.

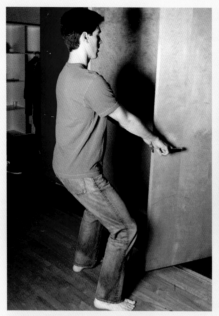

Bend your knees while opposing
the door.

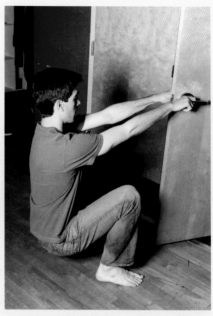

Continue to bend your knees while
opposing the door.

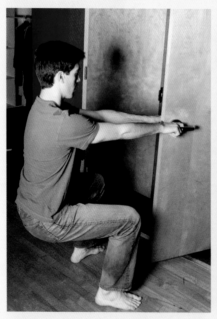

Straighten your knees while opposing
the door.

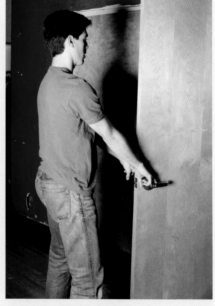

Continue to straighten your knees while
opposing the door.

3. Go back to the chair and try sitting and standing, using the oppositional pulls.

The large pattern of oppositional pulls creates a suspension system. Remember, the body is a suspension system, as we examined in the tensegrity concept. This means that each muscle is stretched just a little bit. This stretch creates tone, like the tensegrity structure. As you develop awareness of these oppositions within yourself, you are able to sense the dynamic opposition between yourself and the audience, creating a dramatic tension.

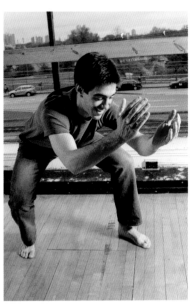

Exploring oppositions.

One acting student observed, "When I did the opposition exercises before I went on stage for *Hamlet*, I felt my body charged and ready to interact with other actors and the audience."

Another student used the opposition idea another way: In her show, Sarah was afraid to display real emotion, because the character she was playing was a prostitute. She said, "I'm holding myself back, but the character does not." I asked her to explore this opposition: to physically move back and forth in space between holding herself back and thrusting her body forward. At first she felt that she, Sarah, was holding back, and the character was enticing her to move forward. However, then it shifted and she felt that she, Sarah, was thrusting herself forward, and the character was retreating back. She felt the opposition between the two. She had discovered a new side of the character that she had not seen before. Her body felt in control, supported, and focused. She then felt ready to display the emotions of a prostitute.

Why I Became an Actor

As I was teaching a group of actors, a question came up, someone in the group asking himself: "Why did I become an actor?" We decided that each student would write a few words about their desire and decision to become an actor.

The answers were varied, honest, and well thought out. "I became an actor because I have an insatiable passion for storytelling." "I want to do everything. I want to be every profession. I am an actor so that I can do everything." "I am an actor because it gives me joy to share a performance with others." As you prepare for a performance, it is sometimes helpful to remember why you chose this profession.

Exercise to Explore "Why I Became an Actor"

Preparation: *Breathe in through the top of your nose to connect your breath with your emotion. Do the Exercise to Explore Monkey or the Exercise to Explore Oppositions, or both, to get your legs flexible and ready to work.*

1. *Remember the first moment you decided to become an actor. What did your body feel like? How did you move around the room? What words did you speak? Explore what it felt like. Move around the room and speak as you did when you first explored acting. Students have said things like, "I can do whatever I want." "I love following my imagination." "I was seven years old and wanted attention."*
2. *Choose a character that you are working on now. Begin to play that character. How does this character move? How does he speak? How does she relate to others? How do you feel as an actor now, playing this role?*
3. *Go back and forth between steps 1 and 2. What are the similarities? What are the differences?*

Students have found: "In step 1, I was never wrong, but in step 2, I became self-conscious." "In step 1, I had this great instinct to play. In step 2, I wondered what was pulling me out of the imaginary circumstances of the play." "I had a similar drive in steps 1 and 2."

As you connect to your own reasons for becoming an actor, bring them to your performance. Remember the joy of sharing your story with others. Remember that you are an artist. Remember the uncensored singing and dancing shows you might have put on as a child. **Bring back some of those exiled parts to create your expanded self or your "new me."**

The Power of Thinking, Feeling, and Sensing, Combined

You saw the link between thoughts and feelings in the Exercise to Explore Inhibition: Chairs, when you moved on every thought from one chair to another. You allowed your body to fill with feelings and sensations before you moved. Or you saw the link in the Exercise to Explore Emotion and Thought, when you thought of an emotion and your partner had to guess it. In chapter 10, "Character and Role," we explored thinking, feeling, and sensing in the triune brain to see the different effects they have in performance. In the following exercise, we will explore how all these elements work together.

Exercise to Explore the Power of Thinking, Feeling, and Sensing, Combined

Preparation: What you think has a great effect on what you do during performance. Recent brain research has shown that when you think about walking, certain areas of the brain light up in a magnetic resonance imaging (MRI) scan. When you actually walk, these same areas light up in the MRI.

To remind you of the power of thinking, stand in a cleared, quiet space. Think the word down. *Continue to think the word* down. *What do you notice in your body? Do the same with the word* up.

1. *Choose one line of text to explore. It may be helpful to choose a line you are having difficulty with.*
2. *Just think your line. Notice what happens.*
3. *Think your line and feel the feelings that go with it. Notice what happens in your body.*
4. *Think, feel, and sense the line. What happens in your body?*
5. *Think, feel, and sense as you speak the line.*
6. *Think, feel, sense, and speak the line as you move in the space.*
7. *Do the piece as yourself, as you would say these words.*
8. *Then do the piece again as your character with only enough white fiber activity to convey the character.*

When you do the line with awareness of thought, feeling, and sensation all at the same time as you speak and move, can you notice a sense of congruence? Your breath, thought, and action are one. Is there fluidity in your body and voice as you speak? Can you feel the freedom to explore, which can inform your performance or shoot?

Performance Preparation

Sometimes before a performance, as preparation, an actor will shake himself or herself, or shake the arms and legs to try to get rid of tension. However, **preparing to perform is not about getting rid of tension, but about redistributing tension, so that it becomes tone.** There is nothing wrong with a little bit of tension. That is what keeps our bodies together. But excess tension can work against you. I call the appropriate amount of tension "tone."

Exercise to Prepare for a Performance

1. *Good preparation is about diving into your body, and noticing what you are doing, thinking, and feeling. With that*

information, you choose what exercises you need to do: the Exercise to Explore Optimal Breath with a Reflex Inhale, the Exercise to Explore Hands on the Back of the Chair, the Exercise to Explore Inhibition: The Three Choices, or others.

2. *Be with what is. If you are angry, figure out how to use that energy to feed the performance.*

3. *Do sound or movement exercises only if it fits your feelings at the moment. There's no need to make random sounds from a class or exercise. Do what is authentic to your needs at the moment.*

4. *To prepare for a performance, you need your ground, your back, your breath, your full stature, and your life force flowing through you, firing away and meeting the room and the life of the play.*

5. *Remember the work in the balance exercise with the example of shifting the chair forward and backward. Now shift yourself forward, back, up, and go.*

I was team-teaching a class with acting professor Judy Braha at Boston University. We were exploring the dynamics of having an acting professor and an Alexander-Movement Specialist in the same room and coaching an actor together to prepare for performance.

One actor felt "stale and out of it." I asked him if he wanted me to put my hands on him. He said "yes," but his body told me "no." So I asked him a few more times. He finally admitted "no," he did not want my hands on. Using the Exercise to Explore "Be With" and the Exercise to Explore a Stuck Place as a model, we explored his state. He said he felt a cement wall around him that was constricting him. The constriction was a clear sign to me that this was an old traumatic response pattern, because there was no reason to have a wall up in this very safe environment, except in his mind and body. I then asked, Might there be a time when the wall need not be up? He said, "At the beach." With that thought, there was less constriction, and his breath began to flow in and out much more freely. Then Judy said, "Can the character also be at the beach?" The cement feeling he'd had changed to a wood feeling, and then eventually dissipated. I then put my hands on him, gently helping guide him in giving his directions. After this, he gave a speech as his character, which brought the audience to tears. It was a command performance.

Exercises to Explore during Performance

1. *Students often ask, "How do I use the Alexander Technique when my character does not have good use?" We talked some about this in regard to the amount of effort you need. In general, when on stage in an uncomfortable position, have a sense of your whole head, in relationship to your whole back, in relationship to your whole body, in relationship to the whole room, and let the ground support you, as you allow micromovements of expansion. Directions are not an end in themselves. Directions allow your neck to be free so that your back can lengthen and widen, so that your life force can move through you. From there you feel the freedom of the opening and allow yourself to transform into the character. After the opening, or the transformation, the directions retreat as background material and become part of your actor self, the same part of yourself that keeps an eye on things like the edge of the stage and where the lights are.*

2. *When you notice people in the audience or on the set and feel anxious, what are you doing to calm yourself down? If you talk to yourself in your head a lot, how could you improve on that? Remember the breathing exercises and the dynamic opposition in yourself and between you and the audience.*

3. *A play is made up of words, sentences, speeches, scenes, acts, and the whole gestalt of the play. It is important to keep the whole life of the play in mind, even as you say a few words.*

4. *Little things keep a performance alive. Follow a small feeling. Let it have its day. What hits you? There is an inner journey. Inner gut feelings are part of it. What happens to you inside when you hear his voice or see her run across the stage? You change. Your body changes. It cannot be the same body moment to moment. Is your body where you are? Let thought live in your body and voice. Find the truth in the moment. Don't lay a wash of artificial neutrality on top.*

5. *In performance, "trying" is not an efficient method. Don't try. Don't hurry. Don't impress. See and deliver. Don't perform. Look at everyone. Be with what is there. Let your eyes look out from the back of your head. This is effortless. See what it is like, not what it should be like. Have a picture and a dramatic imagination. Most characters make a journey within the story of the play. Your dramatic imagination has this journey in mind so you don't need to "try."*

6. *One way to use inhibition when performing is when you notice the audience gets it, take a brief pause. What comes into the space? Allow that in before moving on to the next moment.*

Thomas had a powerful monologue to deliver. He needed to be convincing and strong. He tried hard to force his voice to be emphatic, and his body to be strong. After he did the monologue, I asked him what he noticed. He said he noticed that the monologue went okay, but he felt he was trying too hard. I asked him if his lower legs were involved. He said "no." I asked him to let his lower legs fill with more of himself. After a few moments of this, I asked him to return to the monologue. "Holy cow. I'm just not doing anything, but I can feel so much space. Something really powerful is happening now. This is my moment."

That is what an actor wants to feel during a performance: "This is my moment." I do not mean this to be a puffed-up egoistic concept of yourself, but genuinely giving yourself the time and space to creatively deliver the story.

Exercises to Explore at the End of Performance

At the end of a performance, you must take the time to get the character out of your body, mind, and spirit.

1. *When you finish a performance, if you still feel the emotions of the play and your character gripping your body and mind, take a few minutes to sit and breathe. Try the Exercise to Explore Extending the Exhale: Silent "La La La" and the Exercise to Explore Three-Dimensional Breathing. Do the Exercise to Explore Tracking Your Sensations to calm your nervous system. Or try doing the Exercise to Explore Righting Reflex to Orient Yourself to bring yourself to the present moment.*

2. *If you are still feeling uncomfortable when you get home, take a moment and do the Exercise to Explore Lying-Down Work before you sleep. This can settle your bodily systems and ease your mind.*

One of my students was having nightmares after rehearsing *Marat/Sade*. She tried doing the lying-down work after each show, to acclimate her body back to her daily life, and let the tensions of the play go. Her nightmares subsided.

The thrill of performance for an actor is worth the long hours of preparation, development process, and rehearsal. Your relationship with yourself, the other actors, and the audience comes together to produce the magic of the theater or film. The principles presented in *The Actor's Secret* can help you with the challenges of staying balanced and present to keep this magic alive. The breathing and warm-up exercises can help you with performance preparation and the demands of the theater and the camera. The next chapter will help you meet these demands as you maintain your personal well-being.

CHAPTER 17
Maintaining Health and Well-Being

I was at a master class with Nathan Lane, and one of the students asked him how he maintained such a hectic schedule. He said, **"You need to live like a monk."** Although comic, there is truth to this. Because your body is the instrument you use to convey the story, it must be in good working order. Here are some practices to keep in mind:

1. Eat well.

Eat fresh fruit and vegetables, whole grains and beans, and leaner animal protein, like chicken and fish. Avoid eating large amounts of sugar and refined carbohydrates—the sugar elevates blood sugar levels to spike and then drop down, creating instability in a some-times unstable lifestyle. Also, try not to eat large amounts of dairy because it can create excess mucous, which can hinder your voice. Chewing your food well also helps your digestive system to be able to process food more efficiently and absorb more nutrients.

2. Exercise.

Often the rehearsal process involves some kind of movement warm-up. In addition to that you may require extra effort to keep yourself in tip-top shape. You can swim, bicycle, walk, do yoga or Pilates, or work out. No matter what you choose, you will gain more ben-efit from it if you include the basic directions and pay attention to your use as you exercise. It does not matter so much which type of exercise you choose. It does matter, however, **how** you are doing what you are doing.

3. Get enough rest.

Often actors stay up late because of long hours and late shows. When you come home at night, you might be wound up and need to settle down before sleeping. You need to figure out how much sleep you need to stay healthy and function well. It is different for different people. In order to get enough sleep for your body, you may need to find time for a twenty-minute power nap during the day, or sleep later some mornings.

4. Keep your mind stable by staying with yourself.

This may be the most difficult task. The mind tends to wander. The mind tends to dwell on negative and unproductive thoughts. This can disturb your attention on stage, your sleep patterns, and your health in general. One practice to steady your mind that we have explored is presence—staying aware of the present moment. Also, as we saw in the section on inhibition in chapter 8, meditation can help you stay with yourself in a beneficial way. Meditation teaches your mind to focus on more productive thoughts, and on just being, so that you can deal with whatever thoughts or feelings do arise. One very simple and effective practice is to watch your breathing. Watch the breath come in, and watch the breath go out. If another thought comes in, don't latch on to it and dwell on it, but don't push it away; just continue watching your breath.

In *Hamlet,* Shakespeare wrote, "There is nothing either good or bad, but thinking makes it so." Many actors have anxiety in everyday life. One wonders, "Where will my next role come from, and when?" "How will I pay the rent?" "Am I choosing the right roles?" These questions are very real, but when you think about it, much of the anxiety comes from the mind saying "what if" this happens or "what if" that doesn't happen. When you remain present, calm and centered, you can figure out something that will work for the present moment, which, in reality, is all that exists. The main cause of anxiety is not staying with yourself. When your mind wanders, you leave yourself. You are imagining or fantasizing what might be or who you want to be. You are not present in the here and now to know what is actually happening. When you stay with yourself, you accept all that happens and inquire into it so that you can sort it out. That is not asking for more of the difficult stuff, but it is accepting the truth in the moment. Being with the truth is comforting, even when the truth is unpleasant, because when you have a direct experience of the truth of what is going on, you can choose to do something or to do nothing. But you do enable yourself with having that choice.

Staying with yourself is not the common choice for most people. Many people are influenced by outside circumstances. One young actor, Ken, had just completed an exercise in class. He said, "Betsy asked afterward, 'How does that land on you? What's going on with you right now?' I told her how I honestly felt: 'I can't let in what you've said to me. I'm trying, though.' I breathed, opened up my body, and really tried to let in what she was saying and show it affecting me. To my surprise, Betsy responded, 'Why are you trying? It's okay if you can't let it in,' to which I replied, 'But I don't want to be that scared person.' 'I don't mind seeing scared Ken,' said Betsy. 'But,' I said, 'I don't *want* to be scared Ken.' 'Well why don't you allow your body to do what it wants to do and be who you are, rather than trying to make it do something and be somebody else? **You are denying a part of yourself and trying to be something you're not,**' Betsy said to me. 'You're stopping yourself from being Ken. How does *that* make you feel?' I let go of my 'Alexander-ing' and stopped forcing my body to stay upright and still. I stopped mechanically breathing deeply, and I let my entire torso collapse forward. I began to feel my stomach wring out like a sponge. As if right on cue, Betsy asked, 'What if you sit with that sensation and allow the real Ken to come out? Why don't you be yourself, instead of trying to be something you're not? Sit with that sensation.' I gave in. I let go of control and completely enveloped myself in what I actually wanted to be experiencing. I stopped trying to 'act' in front of Betsy and my peers and stopped suppressing my emotions. While all of this was happening, I began to notice my body lengthening and widening on its own accord. But I wasn't doing anything. Tears were rolling down my cheeks one after another, but I wasn't panting, my face wasn't tense, and I wasn't hysterical at all. It was as if the tears flowed up and out through a clear channel from my gut to my eyes. It was effortless. I felt effortless. But it didn't make any sense—I wasn't doing anything. I felt completely calm and almost peaceful. After class, a classmate came up to me and told me the irony of what had just happened. 'The Ken that you wanted to become and tried to muscle out actually came as a result of sitting with where you were at that moment and allowing yourself to be yourself.'"

This story illustrates that for most of us, when we stop trying to leave ourselves and become what we are not, we give ourselves the chance to become what we are. This is the journey to the physical, mental, emotional, and spiritual expanded self.

THOUGHTS FOR MOVING FORWARD

I have written this book with utter respect, humility, and reverence for the design of the human self, no doubt the most remarkable creation of all. There is so much possibility given to a human being—the ability to choose, to heal, and to change.

As F. M. Alexander was trying to solve his voice problem, he did not know there was a solution to be found. He stumbled on an amazing discovery for human organization and uprightness for health and well-being. Carl Stough found, almost by accident, a coordination for breathing that could heal even emphysema. He found the built-in power of the respiratory mechanism able to heal so deeply. And who would believe that there is a positive side to trauma? Dr. Peter Levine saw that trauma always had another side to it, available for great healing and spiritual growth. By following the body's given cues, listening to the inner messages, there is a way out.

What an amazing design the human body is. Remember the individual stories you saw demonstrated in this book. Remember the two-thousand-pound polar bear who can jump over a cliff as if he weighed practically nothing, or the two-year-old who moves with poise, elegance and grace. Our true nature and design is always there, no matter how many identifications or habits one acquires.

How is your use now as you read this? Have you found your "new me?" Have you realized that the "new me" was always there in you, patiently waiting for you to inhabit by inhibiting, and healing some of your habitual reactions? Your new me just needed a little nudge to emerge and awaken to your expanded self so that you could tell your story as an actor.

Your artistic journey begins the moment you first hold the script in your hand. You have no idea what the future holds or how the artistic process will evolve. After many steps along the way that require flexibility, commitment, discipline, and perseverance, the journey ends with the thrill of the last curtain call, or the last take.

The steps in this book combine the Alexander Technique, Breathing Coordination, and Somatic Experiencing and have the potential to give you a transformative experience on this journey. And what a journey it is! You may have discovered that you can go from "I always feel wrong" to saying "My name is Susan and this is the depth of my voice" in a loud, clear, resonant, unpushed voice. You explored the awareness that "I do not have to be so pulled down and intimidated by that diva on set," and you have balanced a chair and your own weight to find an incredible lightness of body and being. You might have found that you don't need to hold down your emotions with your breath, and now you can fill the four corners of the room with the open-hearted humanity of your character. What a relief to know that holding your legs stiff may actually be an incomplete flight response, and when the response is completed you can run across the stage with ease and fluidity. We explored stuck parts, tight muscles, and held breath, which with awareness and choice you can now transform into tools to help you give a generous command performance.

In this book I have given many exercises to explore and inhibit habitual, surface reactions. After you inhibit your habits that no longer serve you, you can be in touch with a deeper sense of the integrity of your whole being. You can use yourself a different way. You free a pathway for your innate talent to manifest. You are then able to arrive at conscious decisions appropriate for the moment.

The basic principles presented here give you a solid technique to depend on. Allowing your neck to be free immediately opens potential in your throat and voice. Allowing your head to free forward and up brings you to the present moment. Allowing your back to lengthen and widen gives you the strength to bear the truth of the moment. Allowing the ground to support you gives you the relief that you don't need to do it all yourself. "Be with" and tracking your sensations allow you to accept yourself fully. Stop and say "no" to your habitual patterns. This gives you the freedom to reinvent yourself in each moment. These fundamentals provide you with a reliable technique.

After practicing these exercises, you have developed your powers of awareness and observation, released restrictions, increased tone in your musculature, and fine-tuned balance and coordination for effortless movement and presence. You have fuller capacity for breath and life force, and you have freed your voice for communication. With all this, you have the confidence to walk out onto the stage or set and tell your story from the depth of your heart, soul, and being. Do it.

GLOSSARY

directing: The process of sending messages from the brain to the body.

endgaining: Trying to achieve an end result without paying attention to the process or to how the end result is achieved.

faulty sensory perception: What you think you are doing and what you are actually doing may not be the same thing. It is a distortion of the senses.

inhibition: The act of saying "no" to the immediate habitual response so that one can say "yes" to something else.

kinesthetic: One's own sense of movement inside; perception of weight, resistance, and position via the muscular system.

monkey: The term coined by F. M. Alexander's students to describe the position of mechanical advantage, or the ready position.

primary control: Dynamic relationship of neck, head, and back that organizes our movement and alertness.

proprioception: From the Latin *proprio,* meaning "one's own," it is the sense that includes information about what is happening inside your body, such as indicating whether the body is moving with the required effort, and also informing you what is happening at your joints, and where the various parts of the body are located in relation to one another.

reflex: An involuntary, adaptive response to a stimulus.

sensation: Stimulation of an afferent nerve (a nerve going from the body to the brain), changing the state of awareness.

tensegrity: The combination of tension and integrity that demonstrates suspension. The American engineer Buckminster Fuller, who designed the geodesic dome, coined the word.

use: How we use ourselves or how we hold ourselves, including the way the body is shaped, the favored muscular pulls, and how body parts are positioned in relationship to one another.

NOTES

Chapter 1: What Is the Actor's Secret?

1. Edward Maisel, *The Resurrection of the Body* (New York: Dell Publishing, 1969), 2.

Chapter 2: Innovators of Three Somatic Techniques

1. Alexander Techworks website, August 2011, www.alexandertechworks.com/testimonial/sir-ian-mckellen-actor.
2. Carl Stough, *Dr. Breath* (New York: Stough Institute, 1970), 210.
3. Literature for Carl Stough Institute of Breathing Coordination, 1998.
4. Carl Stough, *Breathing: The Source of Life*, DVD video (New York: Stough Institute, 1996).
5. Peter Levine, *Somatic Experiencing Training Course.*

Chapter 4: Five Principles

1. Judy Leibowitz and Bill Connington, *The Alexander Technique* (New York: Harper and Row, 1990), ix.
2. Maisel, 6.
3. F. Matthias Alexander, *The Universal Constant in Living* (New York: E. P. Dutton, 1941), 110.

Chapter 7: Trauma

1. Peter Levine, *In an Unspoken Voice* (Berkeley, CA: North Atlantic Books, 2010), 80.

Chapter 8: Presence and Inhibition

1. Alexander Techworks website, August 2011, www.alexandertechworks.com/testimonial/heath-ledger-actor.
2. Frank Pierce Jones, *Freedom to Change* (London: Mouritz, 1997), 3.
3. Master class with Kevin Spacey at Boston University College of Fine Arts, March 2007.

4. Maisel, 58.

5. Ibid., 4.

6. Levine, *Unspoken Voice*, 129.

Chapter 9: Voice

1. Cornelius L. Reid, *Voice, Psyche and Soma* (New York: Joseph Patelson Music House, 1975), 13.

2. Ibid., 14.

Chapter 13: Monologues

1. Alexander Techworks website, August 2011, http://www.alexander-techworks.com/actor-profile-lynn-redgrave.

2. Personal communication with Sydney Lemmon; used with permission.

3. Steenburgen delivered a talk to the Second International Congress on the F. M. Alexander Technique in Brighton, England, in 1988, as quoted in Direction Journal, http://www.directionjournal.com/brighton-1988.

Chapter 15: Auditions

1. Frank Pierce Jones, *Body Awareness in Action* (New York: Schocken Books, 1976), 132.

2. Levine, *Unspoken Voice*, 146.

3. Master class with Kevin Spacey at Boston University College of Fine Arts, March 2007.

BIBLIOGRAPHY

Alexander, F. Matthias. *Constructive Conscious Control of the Individual.* New York: E.P. Dutton, 1923.

———. *Man's Supreme Inheritance.* New York: E.P. Dutton, 1910.

———. *The Universal Constant in Living.* New York: E.P. Dutton, 1941.

———. *The Use of Self.* New York: E.P. Dutton, 1932.

Caplan, Deborah. *Back Trouble: A New Approach to Prevention and Recovery.* Gainesville, FL: Triad Publishing, 1987.

De Alcantara, Pedro. *Indirect Procedures.* New York: Oxford University Press, 1997.

Garlick, David. *The Lost Sixth Sense: A Medical Scientist looks at the Alexander Technique.* Kensington, Australia: University of New South Wales, 1990.

Gelb, Michael. *Body Learning.* New York: Henry Holt, 1981.

Jones, Frank Pierce. *Body Awareness in Action: A study of the Alexander Technique.* New York: Schocken Books, 1976. Reprinted as *Freedom to Change.* London: Mouritz, 1997.

Herrigel, E. *Zen in the Art of Archery.* New York: Vintage Books, 1971.

Leibowitz, Judy, and Bill Connington. *The Alexander Technique.* New York: Harper and Row, 1990.

Levine, Peter. *In an Unspoken Voice.* Berkeley, CA: North Atlantic Books, 2010.

———. *Waking the Tiger.* Berkeley, CA: North Atlantic Books, 1997.

Maisel, Edward. *The Resurrection of the Body.* New York: Dell, 1969.

———. *Resurrection of the Body: The Essential Writings of F. Matthias Alexander.* New York: University Books, 1989.

Porges, Stephen. *The Polyvagal Theory: Neurophysiological Foundations of Emotions, Attachment, Communication, and Self-Regulation.* New York: W. W. Norton, 2011.

Reid, Cornelius. *Voice, Psyche and Soma.* New York: Joseph Patelson Music House, 1975.

Sherrington, Charles. *The Integrative Action of the Nervous System*. New Haven, CT: Yale University Press, 1961.

Stough, Carl. *Breathing: The Source of Life*. DVD video. New York: Stough Institute, 1996.

———. *Dr. Breath*. New York: The Stough Institute, 1970.

Tinbergen, Nicolas. "Ethology and Stress Disease." *Science* 185 (1974).

INDEX

ABOUT THE AUTHOR

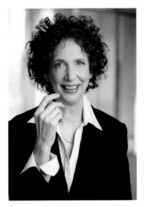

BETSY POLATIN is a movement specialist with four decades of experience in body-mind education and performance training. She has worked with many performing artists in theater, film, and music, including such luminaries as Rashida Jones, Ginnifer Goodwin, Andre Gregory, and John Denver. As a highly respected senior Alexander Technique educator, she pioneered a four-year Alexander curriculum for the acting conservatory program at Boston University's College of Fine Arts, where she is a master lecturer. A certified Breathing Coordination instructor and a Somatic Experiencing practitioner, she holds a BA in dance and an MFA in theater education. She continues to teach her work extensively, both privately and in master classes in the United States and abroad.

About North Atlantic Books

North Atlantic Books (NAB) is an independent, nonprofit publisher committed to a bold exploration of the relationships between mind, body, spirit, and nature. Founded in 1974, NAB aims to nurture a holistic view of the arts, sciences, humanities, and healing. To make a donation or to learn more about our books, authors, events, and newsletter, please visit www.northatlanticbooks.com.

North Atlantic Books is the publishing arm of the Society for the Study of Native Arts and Sciences, a 501(c)(3) nonprofit educational organization that promotes cross-cultural perspectives linking scientific, social, and artistic fields. To learn how you can support us, please visit our website.